Health or Smoking?

4/38

Health or Smoking?

**Follow-up Report of the
Royal College of Physicians**

PITMAN

First Published 1983

Catalogue Number 21.3263.81

Pitman Publishing Ltd
128 Long Acre
London WC2E 9AN

Associated Companies
Pitman Publishing Pty Ltd, Melbourne
Pitman Publishing New Zealand Ltd, Wellington

British Library Cataloguing in Publication Data

Royal College of Physicians of London
　　Health or smoking?: Follow-up report of the
　　Royal College of Physicians of London.
　　1. Tobacco—Physiological effect
　　I. Title
　　613.8′5　　　RA1242.T6
　　ISBN 0-272-79745-6

Printed in Great Britain by
Biddles Ltd, Guildford, Surrey

CONTENTS

THE COMMITTEE

Sir Douglas Black, President (until March, 1983) and Chairman
Dr D J Lane, Hon. Secretary of the Committee
Dr C M Fletcher
Dr D R Harvey
Dr K Horsfield
Dr S P Lock (who also co-edited with the Hon. Secretary)
Dr Celia M Oakley
Dr M P Vessey
Dr D A Pyke, Registrar
Dr D G Williams, Assistant Registrar

Mr G M G Tibbs, College Secretary

Miss K M Snow and Miss L Rathsach, Committee Secretaries

ACKNOWLEDGMENTS

The Committee wishes to acknowledge its indebtedness to the following who, together with committee members, contributed substantially to the text of this report:

Dr Valerie Beral
Mr M Daube
Mr R M Greenhalgh
Dr W W Holland
Dr K D Jamrozik
Dr F Ledwith
Dr P J Lewis
Dr M Murray
Dr R Peto
Dr D J Reid
Dr G A Rose
Mr D Simpson
Dr K B Taylor
Dr N J Wald

Comments on the final text were sought from Sir Richard Doll, Hon. Director Imperial Cancer Research Fund Cancer Unit, University of Oxford, Dr B B Lloyd, recently director of the Health Education Council, and Dr P Sleight, Chairman of ASH.

The College would like to thank the following for permission to reproduce illustrations: British Medical Journal (Figures 3.3, 7.3, 7.4, 8.1) and Lancet (Figure 7.5).

PREFACE

Because of its continuing, and indeed expanding, concern with public health, the Royal College of Physicians has produced a number of reports of Working Parties, on matters as varied as Dietary Fibre, Obesity, Mental Impairment in the Elderly and Death Certification. But in this area of its activities, the College is probably best known to the general public for its reports on the risks to health which arise from the habit of smoking, particularly cigarette smoking, though other forms of smoking are not innocuous, either to the smoker or to his voluntary or involuntary neighbours. The first report, *Smoking and Health*, was published in 1962; the second, *Smoking and Health Now*, in 1971, and the third, *Smoking OR Health*, in 1977.

If this report were merely a recapitulation of the information contained in the three previous reports, there would be little point in issuing it, and indeed we have been careful not to repeat at length points which have become rather generally accepted. But this is an area in which new insights arise, new hazards are discovered or suspected, and new research studies are being made. We have therefore focused major attention on the advances in our understanding of the problems which have occurred in the period since the 1977 report. Thus, we have paid particular attention to the effects of smoking by and on women and children; to the possible risks of passive smoking; to the problem of developing countries; to variation in individual susceptibility to the harmful effects of smoking; and to the opportunities for further initiatives in health education and Government action.

Although some technical language is unavoidable in a serious discussion of the health risks incurred by exposure to tobacco smoke, we have once again tried to express matters simply, and to avoid vain repetition. Sadly, the most repetitive section of the report is that on 'Recommendations' — for the simple reason that so few of those previously made have led to appropriate action on an adequate scale.

Chapter One

INTRODUCTION

Tobacco has been smoked in one form or another in Britain since its introduction here by Raleigh in the reign of the first Elizabeth, and before that had been known to the American Indians for centuries. Up to the late 19th century tobacco was smoked chiefly in pipes and by men. Cigarettes, manufactured for the first time just after the Crimean War, gave a wider public access to tobacco. British men rapidly increased their consumption to an average of 10 cigarettes per adult each day by the time of World War II, and women have followed suit though 40 years later (Figure 1.1) [1]. There has been an encouraging fall in consumption in the last five years and the important part played

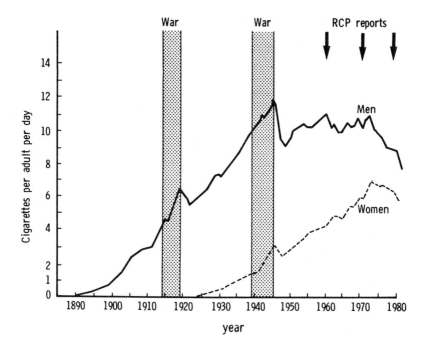

Figure 1.1. Tobacco consumption in the UK 1890 to 1981, given as average number of cigarettes per adult per day for men and women separately, irrespective of whether they smoke or not. The arrows indicate the dates of the three previous Royal College of Physicians reports. Data from Tobacco Research (now Advisory) Council [reference 1 and unpublished data reproduced with permission]

by health education in bringing this about is discussed later in the report (Chapter 11).

Hints that smoking is harmful to health were obtained sporadically many years before the Second World War, but it was not until the 1950s that careful epidemiological studies demonstrated a clear and important association with cancer of the lung [2,3]. Evidence has since emerged of close links between the habit and several other important diseases − among them chronic bronchitis and emphysema [4], coronary heart disease [5] and narrowing of the blood vessels in the limbs [6]; mothers who smoke during pregnancy were found to give birth to smaller babies than mothers who do not smoke and also to have a greater chance of losing their children in the period around birth [7].

The gravity of the health problem created by smoking was highlighted by the first Royal College of Physicians report on smoking in 1962 and underlined by subsequent reports in 1971 and 1977. Yet the problem remains.

At present, tobacco still accounts for some 15 to 20 per cent of all British deaths. Precise calculation is not easy, but with reasonable assumptions the annual death total in the United Kingdom will be not less than 100,000.*

This figure is so large that it completely dwarfs the number of deaths that can be reliably attributed to any other known external factors such as alcohol, road accidents, suicide, etc. Appreciation of the magnitude of the problem is helped by putting the figures in the context of hazards that people already have some feeling for, thus:

Among 1,000 young male adults in England and Wales who smoke cigarettes on average about,

> 1 will be murdered
> 6 will be killed on the roads
> 250 will be killed before their time by tobacco

Besides death must be set the misery to its victims of prolonged ill health, loss of working time and cost to the nation. Sickness due to cigarette smoking leads to the loss of an estimated 50 million working days each year, about four times that due to strikes [8]. The consequent drain on National Health Service resources due to repeated occupancy of hospital beds, sickness benefits and medical care was estimated at £155 million in 1981 [9]. A recent estimate gave the

---

* This figure refers to all ages and is not therefore comparable with mortality figures in previous reports which excluded those over 65 years of age. In 1981 there were about 70,000 deaths from lung cancer, bronchitis and obstructive lung disease, of which at least 90 per cent are attributable to smoking (say 63,000), about 180,000 coronary heart disease deaths, of which perhaps 20 per cent will be related to smoking (say 36,000). These figures together with a few deaths due to miscellaneous other causes related to smoking give a total of over 100,000.

Health or Smoking?: follow up report of the Royal College of Physicians.

Errata (Provisional)

Acknowledgements —   "Dr D J Reid" should be "Mr D J Reid"
Dr B B Lloyd was until recently the Chairman
of the Health Education Council, not its Director.

p 108
The last sentence in the first paragraph should read:
"Estimates based on recent figures suggest that if
the tax percentage on tobacco is kept at its present
level, average consumption of cigarettes per head
of population over 15 years of age will fall by 1999
to 50% of its 1982 value. However if the tax percentage is allowed to rise to maintain Government
revenues from tobacco, then consumption would fall
by 1999 to 30% of the present figures — just over
2 cigarettes per head per day."

p 122 Note 27   "Olsen D V L" should read "Olsen N D L"

cost just of salaries for doctors and nurses caring for patients with smoking-related diseases in Scotland as £6 million [10].

With this vast toll of entirely unnecessary disease and early death it might have been thought that the Government — in view of its avowed "determination to follow a policy aimed at reducing and eventually eliminating the smoking of cigarettes" [11] — would have acted swiftly and in a co-ordinated way to try to prevent what has been called 'the avoidable holocaust'. Sadly, this has been far from the case so that Britain still lags behind several other developed countries in legislation on cigarette smoking. Furthermore, there has been a regrettable tendency to talk of the 'safe cigarette' — a term applied wrongly to one which has a low tar content — and to imply that this is so harmless that the dangers of cigarette smoking have now been overcome. Yet whilst there is now evidence that low tar cigarettes may be responsible for reducing the death rate from lung cancer and possibly other lung diseases (Chapter 3), this is not true for coronary heart disease (Chapter 4) and the risks related to other constituents of cigarette smoke are still present, so perpetuating the public health scandal created by smoking. For these reasons the Royal College of Physicians, which has repeatedly emphasised the dangers of cigarette smoking, has prepared this fourth report: Health *OR* Smoking?

Modern research into the harmful effects of cigarette smoking started from the observation that deaths from lung cancer were rising dramatically. At the beginning of this century this type of cancer was rare, accounting for fewer than 10 deaths in every 100,000 men each year. By 1945, however, the figure had increased tenfold, and by the early 1960s for men aged 45–64 years had peaked at nearly 200 deaths in 100,000 men (Figure 1.2). Today lung cancer is the commonest lethal cancer in Britain.

To explain this dramatic rise in lung cancer deaths, Bradford Hill and Doll started a large-scale inquiry in 1947 [5]. They found that whilst much of the increase in the early years of the century was due to better diagnosis, the more recent increase was chiefly attributable to cigarette smoking. The great majority of all patients had smoked at some time in their lives, but the proportion of smokers was even higher in patients with lung cancer, only a minute proportion of such cases arising in non-smokers. The risks were greater in heavy smokers than in lighter smokers, and cigarette smoking was much more dangerous than either pipe or cigar smoking. These observations were supported by similar studies in other countries [3].

The conclusion that cigarette smoking was responsible for this epidemic was dramatically confirmed by looking at a group of the population that was giving up smoking — doctors. Between 1954 and 1971 the proportion of male doctors smoking cigarettes halved (43% to 21%), while that for all men in England and Wales remained about the same. Over this period the death rate in men from lung cancer fell by 25 per cent in doctors while in the general population it increased by 26 per cent [12].

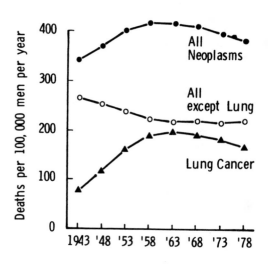

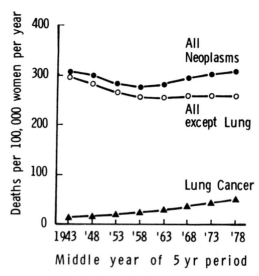

Figure 1.2. Age standardised death rates from all neoplasms, lung cancer and by subtraction all neoplasms other than lung cancer for men and women aged 45–64 years in England and Wales. The recent fall in deaths from lung cancer in men contrasts with the continuing rise in women. For a fuller discussion of these trends see Chapter 3 and Figure 3.1

Apart from cancer of the lung, cancers of the mouth, larynx and oesophagus have all been shown to be associated with smoking and here the risks are as great for pipe and cigar smokers as for those who use cigarettes only. They are, however, less common cancers, and fortunately those in the mouth and larynx are often curable. Less dramatic but still quite clear-cut associations are found between smoking and cancer of the pancreas and cancer of the urinary tract.

The second important condition associated with cigarette smoking is that in which the air passages of the lungs are narrowed and damaged and much of the lung tissue is destroyed. Terminology is complicated. The time-honoured phrase, chronic bronchitis and emphysema, is retained in some sections of this report but reasons for supporting a change of terminology to chronic obstructive lung disease are given in Chapter 3. The condition causes distressing and disabling breathlessness and accounts for an enormous number of days lost from work every year. After prolonged ill health it can prove fatal. Though the death rate has been falling in recent years, still some 20,000 people are certified as dying from this condition in England and Wales every year. Chronic bronchitis and emphysema were until recently known as the 'English disease', and though other factors such as social class and air pollution are partly responsible for their causation, cigarette smoking is now the dominant influence. The death rate from chronic bronchitis is six times as great in smokers as non-smokers, and those smoking over 25 cigarettes a day have 25 times the risk of non-smokers [13]. Recent studies which have further enlarged our understanding of these conditions are discussed in Chapters 3 and 5.

Thirdly, coronary heart disease is now one of the leading causes of death in developed countries. Several factors are recognised as predisposing towards its development, among them heredity, high blood pressure, and possibly a lack of exercise and too much fat in the diet [14]. But strong evidence shows that cigarette smoking also has a profound influence, particularly in people in early middle age. Coronary attacks were shown to be three times as frequent in American men aged 45–54 smoking 15 or more cigarettes a day as in non-smokers [15]. Though the increased risk was less in older men, overall cigarette smoking accounted for about one in three of coronary heart disease deaths. Diseases of the arteries elsewhere than in the heart are also much commoner in smokers than in non-smokers, regular smokers accounting for something like 95 per cent of all patients with serious arterial disease of the legs needing surgical operation [16]. The story of smoking and diseases of the heart and blood vessels is taken up again in Chapter 4.

There is a well recognised association between smoking and peptic ulcers in the stomach and duodenum. Men who smoke have twice as many such ulcers as non-smokers and their ulcers heal poorly and are more likely to lead to a fatal outcome [17]. Several other associations which have been noted in earlier reports remain relatively minor risks besides the main conditions described here.

Finally smoking during pregnancy may put the unborn baby at risk. The implications of smoking in women are considered in detail in Chapter 7 of this report. There is some health risk to children from smoking by their parents and the College remains concerned about the continued uptake of the smoking habit by children and adolescents (see Chapter 6).

A period of some years of smoking is necessary before the increased risk of these conditions becomes apparent. Cigarette smoking was rare until the beginning of this century and became popular among men during World War I, though very few women smoked at this time. In men, cigarette smoking rose steadily to reach a peak in 1945, after which the proportion of men smoking began to fall (detailed prevalence figures for men and women are illustrated in Figure 11.1). It was some 20 years after the smoking habits of men stabilised out that the mortality rates for cancer of the lung also levelled off (Figure 1.2). In women, who started to smoke later and in whom consumption has only recently levelled off, lung cancer deaths continue to rise. The latest trends in lung cancer mortality are of considerable interest and the subject of more detailed discussion later in this report (Chapters 3 and 5). Mortality from chronic bronchitis and emphysema has tended to fall very gradually and did not in the early years of this century show any rise that paralleled the rise in cigarette consumption. It seems likely that this is due first to enormous problems with disease classification, and secondly to a concurrent decrease in mortality following a reduction in other causes of the disease. Mortality rates for coronary heart disease were static in Britain until very recently, though significant falls had already been noted in the USA, Australia, Belgium and a few other countries [18]. Several factors other than smoking play a part in the causation of coronary heart disease, making the quantitative role of cigarette smoking more difficult to determine.

Are there any 'benefits' of smoking? Smokers tend to be thinner than non-smokers. Among men over 40 working in the steel industry the smokers were on average seven per cent lighter than the non-smokers [19]. Despite this, smokers die at a younger age than non-smokers, and non-smoking men require to be 35 per cent overweight (50% in women) before they have the same mortality risk as smokers of normal weight [20]. Furthermore, loss of weight in middle-aged smokers could point to deteriorating lung function rather than any benefit from smoking [19]. There are slight but definite personality differences between smokers as a group, who tend to be more extroverted than non-smokers, but it seems likely that this is a personality trait that is associated with the tendency to take up cigarette smoking rather than being a 'beneficial' effect of smoking itself. Nevertheless, it has been shown that there are a few illnesses which smokers are less liable to develop than are non-smokers; among these are toxaemia of pregnancy [21], pulmonary embolus after operation [22], Parkinson's disease

[23] and possibly ulcerative colitis [24]. It must be emphasised, however, that in all cases the risks of regular cigarette smoking are vastly greater than are these minor benefits.

In committed smokers the purpose of the habit seems to be to deliver regular doses of nicotine to the brain, where it can cause complex and apparently paradoxical effects, such as arousal or sedation, and improvement or worsening of concentration. Understanding of the smoker's perceived need for nicotine has progressed considerably in recent years and a subsequent section of this report (Chapter 2) will discuss how this leads the smoker to regulate his intake – so that after switching to low tar cigarettes he may smoke more, take more puffs per cigarette, or inhale more deeply. Opposing this need, however, are factors such as expense and risk to health. Although about 70 per cent of smokers make one or more attempts to stop, only 20 per cent of regular smokers eventually succeed in doing so, though, contrary to popular belief, only 14 per cent of those who do succeed find it very difficult. The doctors in Bradford Hill and Doll's study who gave up smoking reported more advantages than disadvantages, being less tense or irritable and more energetic than previously. Firm, direct but individual counselling appears to be as effective as complex methods in achieving this goal.

The six years that have elapsed since the last College report have seen the virtual rejection by the smoking public of cigarettes containing tobacco substitutes. This may be no bad thing, as the part-substitute brands marketed in 1977 produced about as much tar as other brands then currently on the market. Brands of cigarettes giving low tar yields may, by contrast, really be somewhat less dangerous and this issue is considered in Chapter 9. They should not, however, be looked upon as 'safe'.

In the past two or three years attention has been focused on the possible hazards of 'passive' smoking – that is, breathing in other people's tobacco smoke. Formerly any true hazards to health from passive smoking (other than for children) had been dismissed as relatively rare; an occasional person might be truly allergic to tobacco smoke, developing asthma if exposed to it, but in most the problem was irritation of the eyes, nose and throat, and headache. Recent research has, however, suggested that the non-smoker inhaling other people's smoke may be at some small risk from health hazards similar to those which affect smokers, although at present much of the evidence is inconclusive. Other studies have shown that passive smoking can be harmful to those with heart and lung disease and underline the basic right of the non-smokers to work, eat and play in non-polluted atmospheres. This important topic is the subject of a separate chapter in this report (Chapter 8).

Faced with such an enormous problem in public health – comparable with that of the devastating epidemics of infectious disease of the past – the health professions have consistently given advice to the public and have made recommendations to Government about what action should be taken.

The Chief Medical Officer of the Department of Health has repeatedly emphasised the true costs to the community of cigarette smoking, and in 1968 the DHSS set up the Health Education Council and the Scottish Health Education Unit. The organisation ASH (Action on Smoking and Health) was established by the Royal College of Physicians in 1971 to co-ordinate voluntary efforts against smoking and has subsequently acted as an important pressure group. The College has issued three reports (1962, 1971 and 1977), the last of which drew up seven recommendations for action:

A rigorous public education programme, particularly aimed at encouraging children not to smoke

Measures in the National Health Service, including limiting smoking in hospitals and elsewhere;

Restrictions on smoking in public places;

Phasing out of tobacco sales promotion;

Differential price rises for tobacco products discriminating against the high tar/nicotine cigarette;

Withdrawal of high tar/nicotine cigarettes as soon as possible;

A large increase in research, possibly with the creation of a special smoking research unit.

Only one of these measures — differential taxation of the highest tar yielding cigarettes — was put into effect. Regrettably the Supplementary Tar Tax was withdrawn in 1981, though fortunately average tar yields of British cigarettes have continued to fall (see Chapter 2). As to the others, there has either been no real action or even the reverse — the virtual go-ahead to the tobacco manufacturers to proceed with direct advertising, sponsorship, or other schemes to encourage the sale of their products. Thus currently the tobacco industry is spending £100 million annually on promoting its products, compared with the grant of £145,000 to ASH and of £8.5 million to the Health Education Council and £2 million to the Scottish Health Education Group (which are, of course, also concerned with many projects other than discouraging cigarette smoking). Health Ministers known to favour the prevention programme were moved to other departments in the Government following tough negotiations with the industry over the abolition of voluntary agreements on sales promotion. No effective Government action has been taken to reduce and eventually abolish advertising — though experience in other countries, such as Norway and Finland, that have strict tobacco acts forbidding advertising has suggested that such measures can affect the proportion of children who start to smoke. Finally, against advice from bodies concerned with health, the Government has allowed the tobacco industry to attempt to gain some credibility by allocating money for research into health, yet with the exclusion of research related to smoking cessation.

It is small wonder then – at a time when national institutions, such as opera houses, theatres and orchestras, as well as sporting events, are increasingly relying on sponsorship from tobacco companies (and in doing so circumventing the Government ban on television advertising) – that all these failures on the part of successive Governments to take action to curb a lethal habit have angered and depressed those concerned for the public health. Government has a responsibility both to inform and to act – not only to warn of health dangers but to legislate for the good of the individual and the community. These issues are taken up again in Chapter 11, and the wider responsibilities of this nation to try to prevent the spread of the smoking habit in the developing world are the subject of special attention in Chapter 10.

Smoking still kills, and at a time when some 100,000 of our citizens are dying prematurely from its effects every year and millions more will die elsewhere, the Royal College of Physicians would be failing in its duty if it did not urge the Government to reverse its present attitude of inactivity and even of encouragement towards the tobacco industry and tackle this hidden holocaust with the urgency once given to cholera, diphtheria, poliomyelitis and tuberculosis. Our recommendations for ways of achieving this form the final chapter of the report (Chapter 12).

References

1   Lee PN, ed. *Statistics of Smoking in the United Kingdom, 7th Edition.* Tobacco Research Council Research Paper 1. 1976
2   Doll R, Hill AB. A study of the aetiology of carcincoma of the lung. *Br Med J 1952; 2:* 1271–1276
3   World Health Organization. Epidemiology of cancer of the lung. Report of a study group. *WHO Tech Rep Ser 1960:* 192
4   Anderson DO, Ferris BG. Role of tobacco smoking in the causation of chronic respiratory disease. *N Engl J Med 1962; 267:* 787–794
5   Doll R, Hill AB. Mortality in relation to smoking: ten years' observation of British doctors. *Br Med J 1964; 1:* 1399–1410, 1460–1467
6   Larson PS, Haag HB, Silvette H. *Tobacco: Experimental and Clinical Studies. A Comprehensive Account of the World Literature.* Baltimore: Williams & Wilkins. 1961
7   Butler NR, Alberman ED, eds. *Perinatal Problems: The Second Report of the British Perinatal Mortality Survey.* Edinburgh: E & S Livingstone. 1969
8   Bow Group Memorandum. *A Healthier Future.* March 1980: 3
9   Finsberg G (43rd Series). *(26 January 1982); 16:* col. 337. London: Hansard
10 Brotherston KG. *The Scottish Epidemic.* ASH Scottish Committee of Action on Smoking and Health. 1982
11 HC Debate (5th Series). *(9 July 1979); 970:* col. 49. London: Hansard
12 Doll R, Peto R. Mortality in relation to smoking: twenty years' observations of British doctors. *Br Med J 1976; 4:* 1525–1536
13 Royal College of Physicians. *Smoking and Health Now: 2nd Report.* London: Pitman. 1971
14 Reid DD, Hamilton PJS, McCartney P et al. Smoking and other risk factors for coronary heart disease in British civil servants. *Lancet 1976; ii:* 979–984

15   US Department of Health Education and Welfare. *The Health Consequences of Smoking. A Report to the Surgeon General.* DHEW Publication No (HSM) 71-7513. 1971

16   Begg TB. Characteristics of men with intermittent claudication. *Practitioner 1965; 194:* 202–207

17   Friedman GD, Siegelaub AB, Seltzer CC. Cigarettes, alcohol, coffee and peptic ulcer. *N Engl J Med 1974; 290:* 469–473

18   World Health Organization Regional Office for Europe. *Myocardial Infarction Community Registers.* Published annually Copenhagen

19   Nemery B, Moavero NE, Brasseur L, Stanescu DC. Smoking, lung function, and body weight. *Br Med J 1983; 386:* 249–251

20   Lew EA, Garfinkel L. Variations in mortality by weight among 750,000 men and women. *J Chron Dis 1979; 32:* 563–576

21   Palmgren B, Wahlen T, Wallander B. Toxaemia and cigarette smoking during pregnancy: prospective consecutive investigation of 3,927 pregnancies. *Acta Obstet Gynecol Scand 1973; 52:* 183–185

22   Clayton JK, Anderson JA, McNicol GP. Effect of cigarette smoking on subsequent post-operative thromboembolic disease in gynaecological patients. *Br Med J 1978; 2:* 402

23   Godwin-Austen RB, Lee PN, Marmot MG, Stern GM. Smoking and Parkinson's Disease. *J Neurol Neurosurg Psychiatry 1982; 45:* 577–582

24   Jick H, Walker AM. Cigarette smoking in ulcerative colitis. *N Engl J Med 1983; 308:* 261–263

Chapter Two

THE PHARMACOLOGY AND TOXICOLOGY
OF TOBACCO SMOKING

SMOKE AND SMOKING

The average British filter tip cigarette is smoked in nine or ten puffs over 10 minutes. With each puff the smoker draws air through the burning tip of the cigarette and about 50ml of smoke enters the mouth. This intake of smoke contains about 50mg of material, 18mg of which is solid particulate matter [1]. The rest consists of gases and vapourised materials, of which up to five per cent is the toxic gas carbon monoxide. The particulate material in the smoke is an aerosol of tar in which the alkaloid drug nicotine is dissolved. The tar is so finely dispersed that each droplet is only half a micron in diameter, less than one ten thousandth of the size of a pin head. A single cigarette delivers to the smoker a million million of these tiny particles [1]. As the cigarette burns down so the concentration of tar and carbon monoxide in the smoke increases.

Once the smoke is in the mouth, most cigarette smokers take a breath and inhale it into the air passages and so down into the lungs. With the next breath some smoke is exhaled. However, appearances are deceptive: inhaling cigarette smokers breathe out only a small proportion of the smoke they inhale [2]. All the carbon monoxide, over 90 per cent of the nicotine and 70 per cent of the tar are retained. Whilst tar particles in the smoke are deposited in the airways, the nicotine diffuses into the blood, rapidly reaching the brain, where it exerts the pharmacological effects which are thought to form the habituating basis of the tobacco smoking habit.

Smoking is thus an extremely rapid, simple and efficient process. The desired drug, nicotine, is transferred from the tobacco leaf to its site of action in the brain in less than 30 seconds. However, during the process the body takes in many other toxic substances. Previous College reports have detailed the evidence concerning the harmful effects of tars, which are largely responsible for lung cancer, and irritant substances, which may cause chronic bronchitis, as well as giving information on the known effects of nicotine and carbon monoxide [3].

Some recent evidence concerning the toxicity of cigarette smoke in relation to lung cancer and chronic obstructive lung disease is discussed in Chapters 3 and 5 and the controversial issue of the importance of carbon monoxide for diseases of the circulation is raised in Chapter 4. This chapter will concentrate chiefly on nicotine. There has been for some time strong support for the view that smoking is both pleasurable and addictive on account of the nicotine content of cigarette smoke. Recent reports have, however, cast some doubts on this view and this section will consider the evidence.

NICOTINE

Nicotine, an alkaloid, is a naturally occurring drug which is present in a concentration of up to three per cent by weight in the tobacco plant. Most of the nicotine survives the smoking process intact and each puff of cigarette smoke enables the inhaling smokers to absorb between 0.1 and 0.2mg of nicotine, the average sales-weighted nicotine delivery of UK cigarettes in 1981 being 1.33mg. The concentration of nicotine in the blood rises steeply during smoking and reaches a peak just after the last puff, when the concentration can vary between 10 and 40µg/litre [4]. In cigar smokers the level in the blood may be higher − up to 65µg/litre [2].

Nicotine is toxic if administered in large doses. To swallow a single dose of 60mg is said to be fatal to the average man. A cigarette yields much less than this, under 2mg, and smokers are more tolerant to the toxic effects of nicotine than non-smokers. Few toxic effects can be demonstrated in animals when they are given small doses of nicotine over long periods of time, mimicking the intake of smokers.

In man several effects of nicotine are now well described.

Subjective effects

Once habituated most smokers report that smoking induces a feeling of relaxation. Situations of stress are apparently faced more easily and boring tasks carried out more efficiently. Conversely when nicotine or smoking is withdrawn smokers become unduly irritable, a withdrawal reaction [5].

Cardiovascular effects

Nicotine increases heart rate and blood pressure. The effects are produced by the drug stimulating the autonomic nerves which control heart rate and constriction in blood vessels, and also by the release of adrenaline from the adrenal glands [6]. Nicotine also increases the stickiness of blood platelets [7]. As a consequence nicotine can make existing peripheral vascular disease more severe and, in patients with established heart disease, can precipitate an episode of irregular heart beat [8: see also Chapter 4]. The cardiovascular effects of nicotine are most marked following the first cigarette of the day, relative tolerance developing as continued smoking builds up the level of nicotine [9].

Alimentary tract

Nausea and vomiting are induced by high doses of nicotine in smokers and by only small doses in non-smokers who are not habituated to nicotine. Tolerance to this effect occurs if the novice smoker persists with the habit. Nicotine also increases the mobility of the bowel, which affects the speed of food transit and increases gastric acid secretion, thus promoting the development of peptic ulcers.

On the other hand, nicotine appears not to be carcinogenic of itself, though there is evidence that it may enhance the carcinogenic effects of benzo-a-pyrene, one of the most dangerous components of cigarette tar [10]. Thus, nicotine is relatively non-toxic when compared with many other components of tobacco smoke. It is perhaps ironic that smokers are being poisoned not by the drug they are smoking for but by impurities they take in with it.

Nicotine dependence

Whilst smoking behaviour clearly demonstrates all the features of a habit, there is little doubt too that smokers derive pleasure from smoking, and persist with their habit in order to satisfy their need for these pleasurable sensations. They thus become dependent on or addicted to smoking.*

Several lines of evidence suggest that the most likely dependence-inducing substance amongst the several thousand chemicals in tobacco smoke is nicotine [11]. As described above, smokers develop tolerance to the physiological effects of nicotine. Furthermore, they feel unwell if they stop smoking and their withdrawal symptoms can be abolished with nicotine. Tolerance and withdrawal symptoms are classic features of drug dependence. Nicotine-free cigarettes made from lettuce or artificial materials have never achieved popularity. Indeed only materials which yield active drugs are sought after by large numbers of people for smoking or inhaling, and tobacco is one of a short list of such substances which includes opium, cocaine and hashish.

If nicotine is truly the addictive component in cigarette smoke, then when the amount of nicotine delivered by cigarettes is reduced, smokers should respond by smoking more intensely. Equally it should be possible to satisfy the smoker's need for nicotine by administering the drug in ways other than smoking.

Smokers certainly change the way in which they smoke when given cigarettes that yield different amounts of nicotine, tar and carbon

---

* The World Health Organization in 1964 recommended that the term drug addiction be replaced by drug dependence − a compulsion to continue taking a drug in order to experience its mental effects or to avoid the discomfort caused by abstinence from the drug.

monoxide [12,13]. Bearing in mind that measurements of yield from cigarettes are determined from experiments using smoking machines, and that these may well not match yields obtained by actual smokers, most studies suggest that smokers can detect the 'strength' of a cigarette. Cigarettes with a low tar/nicotine yield are perceived by smokers as 'weak' and they have a strong tendency to puff such low nicotine cigarettes more frequently, to inhale more deeply and to smoke to a shorter butt length [14].

Do these changes in smoking pattern compensate for the reduction in nicotine yield per cigarette? Some studies certainly suggest that they do: others do not. At one extreme, in a study of blood nicotine concentrations in 300 smokers attending a smoking withdrawal clinic, very little difference was found in average concentrations between smokers of high, medium and low nicotine cigarettes [15]. Hence these smokers tended to compensate almost completely for the different deliveries of their cigarettes so as to maintain their accustomed concentration of blood nicotine. These smokers, however, were seeking help in stopping smoking by attending an anti-smoking clinic and may have been highly addicted to cigarettes and therefore not a random sample of smokers. At the other extreme, there are studies which show that compensation is often not complete. Three studies report no change at all in cigarette consumption after decreases in nicotine yield of 20 to 30 per cent.

At least 18 studies have been made of changes in cigarette consumption when cigarette smokers are given higher or lower nicotine cigarettes to smoke. In some of these studies the period of observation has been a few days, in others many months, but to take all studies together, it appears that, on average, smokers increase their cigarette consumption only by about 10 per cent for as much as a 50 per cent decrease in nicotine delivery [16].

There has been a natural experiment in changing nicotine yields from manufactured cigarettes in that, over the period 1969–1973, average nicotine delivery fell by 32 per cent from 1.76 to 1.33mg per cigarette. At the same time the annual number of cigarettes consumed per smoker in Britain rose by about 18 per cent in both men and in women (Figure 2.1). This is a much greater degree of compensation than the studies summarised above would indicate, but the changes in consumption are influenced by many other factors, not least of which is cost. Over this period of rising consumption, the real cost of cigarettes fell (see Chapter 11). Furthermore, if those who stopped smoking over the period were lighter smokers than average, consumption in those who continued to smoke would appear to increase [17].

A fundamental problem with all these studies is that together with a reduction in nicotine yields there has also been a reduction in tar and, to some extent, carbon monoxide yields (see Figure 9.1). Tar is probably the more important, for undoubtedly much of the flavour or 'scratch' which contributes to the smoker's detection of the strength

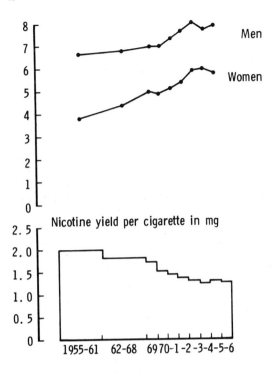

Figure 2.1. Average sales-weighted nicotine delivery of cigarettes marketed in the United Kingdom from 1955 to 1976 with annual consumption of cigarettes in thousands plotted separately for men and women. Over this period as the nicotine yield declined so consumption increased

of cigarettes, and perhaps gives pleasure, is due to the tar content. Detailed experiments in which tar and nicotine yields have been varied independently are few, but of great interest.

When two high tar cigarettes were compared, one with medium nicotine and the other low nicotine, subjects certainly took smaller puffs from the cigarettes yielding more nicotine and also took in less smoke as judged by carbon monoxide intake [18]. In another study where two low tar cigarettes yielding either medium or low nicotine were compared, few differences emerged except that those smokers who previously had been accustomed to smoking medium tar cigarettes oversmoked the low tar cigarettes irrespective of their nicotine content [19]. This suggests that they were attemping to compensate for the lower tar yield rather than for the nicotine. Further support for this came from a study of 55 smokers allowed to smoke their usual brand of cigarettes [20]. Irrespective of the nicotine yield of the cigarettes, smokers of lower tar cigarettes puffed more smoke in an apparent attempt to increase the amount of tar inhaled.

Studies in which nicotine is administered to smokers by routes other than inhaling also give some confusing results. It would be expected that if the need for nicotine is already supplied, smokers would smoke fewer cigarettes. Nicotine injected over six hours up to the equivalent of about 17 cigarettes did lead to a 30 per cent reduction in cigarettes smoked [21], but attempts to mimic the fluctuating blood concentrations produced by smoking with intermittent injections did not result in any reduction in cigarette consumption [22].

Until recently direct injection into the blood appeared to be the only way of administering nicotine which is as effective as smoking in raising the blood level of nicotine rapidly. However, recently it has been shown that nicotine snuff gives a pattern of absorption exactly like that of cigarette smoking and this may prove to be a useful tool in investigating the role of nicotine in cigarette dependence [23].

If nicotine is swallowed, it is absorbed from the stomach but broken down by the liver before reaching high levels in circulating blood. However, if nicotine is chewed in the mouth, then sufficient can be absorbed into the blood to satisfy some of the craving for nicotine. This fact has long been known. Sailors in Nelson's day, who were not allowed to smoke while on duty, chewed tobacco. Today, nicotine impregnated chewing gum has been used with some success in weaning smokers off their habit when administered as part of an overall smoking withdrawal programme [24]. Results of the latest trials suggest that the usefulness of this approach in general practice without other reinforcement to give up smoking is limited [25], indicating again that there is more to the smoking habit than simply nicotine dependence.

Psychological dependence

To emphasise the role of nicotine in producing dependence or addiction leaves aside other evidence regarding the psychological uses of smoking, though even here the effect may be mediated by nicotine. As pointed out above, smoking has effects on behaviour that are apparently conflicting, being capable of both producing relaxation and increasing efficiency. The electrical activity of the brain has been shown to be activated by smoking in a number of experiments [26]. However, if the smoker is highly stressed by being exposed to bursts of intense noise, then smoking a cigarette decreases brain activation [27]. This type of result has echoes in studies which record increased smoking under conditions of stress, such as watching horrifying films [28]. On the other hand, in circumstances where a monotonous task is being carried out which requires considerable vigilance, smoking increases arousal, and leads to a maintained efficiency beyond that seen in smokers deprived of cigarettes [29] or in non-smokers performing the same task [30]. No direct evidence in man points to nicotine as the agent in cigarette smoke responsible for these psychological effects, but in animals nicotine can certainly cause arousal [31], reduce aggressive behaviour [32] and lessen the effects of stress [33].

Whilst these studies are certainly far from giving a complete picture of the nature of cigarette dependence, they do suggest that the smokers' claims that smoking helps to maintain attention in the performance of boring routines and helps them cope with stress, are valid and important. The recognition of this makes any understanding of the smokers' desire to smoke much easier but renders the task of helping smokers to give up much more complex.

CARBON MONOXIDE AND SMOKING HABITS

Cigarette smoke contains up to five per cent carbon monoxide and the average current sales-weighted carbon monoxide delivery for British cigarettes is 16.6mg. Though the yield of carbon monoxide has declined a little over the last 40 years, this is not so obvious as the changes in tar and nicotine (see Figure 9.1). Reductions in carbon monoxide yield do not necessarily accompany reductions in tar and nicotine and indeed it will be impossible to eliminate carbon monoxide altogether because it is an inevitable by-product of combustion.

The carbon monoxide concentration of cigarette smoke varies according to how closely the tobacco is packed, the type of paper used in the cigarette, whether the filter is ventilated and the length of the unsmoked butt. If the tobacco is loosely packed and holes are made in the filter, this reduces the carbon monoxide concentration. However, these ventilation holes in the filter also make the cigarette draw poorly and it has been shown that smokers may adjust their smoke intake to get around this, by blocking the aeration holes in the filter. Sometimes the smoker does this unconsciously by closing his lips around the holes, sometimes by pinching the filter, and smokers may even wrap sticky tape around cigarette filters to get a more satisfying smoke [34]. At the same time the carbon monoxide yield from the cigarette will rise. One smoking strategy which reduces total carbon monoxide yield is to leave long unsmoked butts whilst compensating by smoking more cigarettes [35]. This is, of course, an expensive option and British smokers tend to smoke to shorter butt lengths than do smokers in the United States.

Carbon monoxide is toxic [36], exerting its deleterious effects by reducing the oxygen-carrying capacity of the blood (see further Chapter 4). However, despite the above comments of altered smoking behaviour with filter cigarettes, there is no suggestion that carbon monoxide is implicated in cigarette dependence.

A PHARMACOLOGICAL APPROACH TO SMOKING CESSATION

Deaths from smoking-related diseases will be reduced only if smokers smoke less, if smoking becomes less dangerous or if fewer people smoke. The primary aim has always been to persuade people not to smoke by informing them of the risks that they run. However, to the average smoker the risks are remote whilst the satisfaction is immediate. As a consequence, over one-third of adults in Britain continue to smoke. How can a knowledge of pharmacology help to change this?

In the first place, pharmacology suggests that for some smokers the smoking habit is far from being under rational control by the smoker. These smokers are habituated, addicted or dependent on nicotine or conceivably to some other component of cigarette smoke. They have a strong compulsion to continue to smoke. Stopping smoking is physically unpleasant. This means quitting smoking is not necessarily the trivial exercise of willpower that a lot of non-smokers imagine it to be, and it may be a very difficult task which the smoker needs help to complete. Secondly, it seems that nicotine may be the component in cigarettes that lies behind the psychological support that other smokers obtain from smoking in situations of stress or boredom. Pharmacology also gives some guidance on the mode of giving up smoking that is most likely to be effective. If nicotine is a major factor in cigarette dependence then the use of nicotine by other routes, for example in chewing gum, to substitute for smoking could be effective and would be rational. If on the other hand some component of cigarette tar is responsible for cigarette dependence, then the task of helping the would be ex-smoker by providing tobacco substitutes is very much greater.

These arguments are central to the issue of less hazardous smoking. This important topic is discussed later in this report (Chapter 9). Present knowledge suggests that no cigarette can ever be completely safe. Some of the evidence suggests that a cigarette which yielded a dose of nicotine high enough to satisfy the smoker whilst producing a minimal yield of tar and carbon monoxide would be the answer. If on the other hand further research supports the view that tar is also implicated, this answer will not satisfy the dependent smokers, and if other studies point to more harm from nicotine than is at present evident, this answer will not satisfy the urgent need to reduce the death toll from smoking-related diseases.

References

1   Wald N, Doll R, Copeland G. Trends in tar, nicotine, and carbon monoxide yields of UK cigarettes manufactured since 1934. *Br Med J 1981; 282:* 763–766
2   Armitage A, Dollery CT, Houseman T et al. Absorption of nicotine from small cigars. *Clin Pharmacol Ther 1978; 23:* 143–151
3   Royal College of Physicians. *Smoking Or Health: 3rd Report.* Tunbridge Wells: Pitman Medical. 1977
4   Armitage AK, Dollery CT, George CF et al. Absorption and metabolism of nicotine from cigarettes. *Br Med J 1975; 4:* 313–316
5   Lader M. Nicotine and smoking behaviour. *Br J Clin Pharmacol 1978; 5:* 289–292

6   Tachmes L, Fernandez RJ, Sackner MA. Hemodynamic effects of smoking cigarettes of high and low nicotine content. *Chest 1978; 74:* 243–246

7   US Public Health Service. *The Health Consequences of Smoking.* Supplement to Public Health Service Publication No 1696. 1968: 34

8   Herxheimer A, Griffiths RL, Hamilton B, Wakefield M. Circulatory effects of nicotine aerosol inhalation and cigarette smoking in man. *Lancet 1967; ii:* 754–755

9   Jarvik ME. Tolerance to the effects of tobacco. *Natl Inst Drug Abuse Res Monogr Ser 1979; 23:* 150–157

10   Bayne CK. *A Probability Prediction Model of Mouse Skin Tumours Based on Chemical Components of Cigarette Smoke Condensates.* Oak Ridge, Tennessee: US Department of Energy, Oak Ridge National Laboratory. Publication No ORNL/TM-7037. 1979: 38

11   Kumar R, Lader M. Nicotine and smoking. *Curr Dev Psychopharmacol 1981; 6:* 127–164

12   Freedman S, Fletcher CM. Changes of smoking habits and cough in men smoking cigarettes with 30% NSM tobacco substitute. *Br Med J 1976; 1:* 1427–1430

13   Guillerm R, Radziszewski E. Analysis of smoking pattern including intake of carbon monoxide and influence of changes in cigarette design. In Thornton RE, ed. *Smoking Behaviour: Physiological and Psychological Influences.* Edinburgh: Churchill Livingstone. 1978

14   Henningfield JE, Griffiths RR. Effects of ventilated cigarette holders on cigarette smoking by humans. *Psychopharmacology 1980; 68:* 115–119

15   Russell MAH, Jarvis M, Iyer R, Feyerabend C. Relation of nicotine yield of cigarettes to blood nicotine concentrations in smokers. *Br Med J 1980; 280:* 972–976

16   Stepney R. Consumption of cigarettes of reduced tar and nicotine delivery. *Br J Addict 1980; 75:* 81–85

17   Ashton M, Stepney R. *Smoking: Psychology and Pharmacology.* London: Tavistock Publications. 1982

18   Herning RI, Jones RT, Bachman J, Mines AH. Puff volume increases when low-nicotine cigarettes are smoked. *Br Med J 1981; 283:* 187–189

19   Stepney R. Would a medium-nicotine, low tar cigarette be less hazardous to health? *Br Med J 1981; 283:* 1292–1296

20   Sutton SR, Russell MAH, Iyer R et al. Relationship between cigarette yields, puffing patterns and smoke intake: evidence for tar compensation? *Br Med J 1982; 285:* 600–603

21   Lucchesi BR, Schyster CR, Emley GS. The role of nicotine as a determinant of cigarette smoking frequency in man with observations of certain cardiovascular effects associated with the tobacco alkaloid. *Clin Pharmacol Ther 1967; 8:* 789–794

22   Kumar R, Cooke EC, Lader MH, Russell MAH. Is nicotine important to tobacco smoking? *Clin Pharmacol Ther 1977; 21:* 520–529

23   Russell MAH, Jarvis MJ, Feyerabend C, Fernö O. Nasal nicotine solution: a potential aid to giving up smoking? *Br Med J 1983; 286:* 683–684

24   Russell MAH, Raw M, Jarvis MJ. Clinical use of nicotine chewing-gum. *Br Med J 1980; 280:* 1599–1602

25   Research Committee of the British Thoracic Society: report by a subcommittee. Comparison of four methods of smoking withdrawal in patients with smoking related diseases. *Br Med J 1983; 286:* 595–597

26   Knott VJ, Venables PN. EEG Alpha correlates of non-smokers, smokers, smoking and smoking deprivation. *Psychophysiology 1977; 14:* 150–156

27   Mangan GL, Golding J. An 'enhancement' model of smoking maintenance? In Thornton RE, ed. *Smoking Behaviour: Physiological and Psychological Influences.* Edinburgh: Churchill Livingstone. 1978

28   Frith CD. Smoking behaviour and its relation to the smoker's immediate experience. *Br J Soc Clin Psychol 1971; 10:* 73–78

29   Frankenhauser M, Myrsten A-L, Post B, Johansson G. Behavioural and physiological effects of cigarette smoking in a monotonous situation. *Psychopharmacologia 1971; 22:* 1–7

30   Wesnes K, Warburton DM. The effects of cigarette smoking and nicotine tablets upon human attention. In Thornton RE, ed. *Smoking Behaviour.* Edinburgh: Churchill Livingstone. 1978: 131–147

31   Domino EF. Electroencephalographic and behavioural arousal effects of small doses of nicotine: a neuropsychopharmacological study. *Ann NY Acad Sci 1967; 142:* 216–244

32   Hutchinson RR, Emley GS. Effects of nicotine on avoidance, conditioned suppression and aggression response measures in animals and man. In Dunn WL, ed. *Smoking Behaviour: Motives and Incentives.* Washington DC: Winston. 1973

33   Nelsen JM. Psychological consequences of chronic nicotinisation: a focus on arousal. In Battig K, ed. *Behavioural Effects of Nicotine.* Basel: Karger. 1978

34   Kozlowski LT, Frecker RC, Khouw V, Pope MA. The misuse of 'less-hazardous' cigarettes and its detection: hole blocking of ventilated filters. *Am J Public Health 1980; 70:* 1202–1203

35   Marcus AH, Czajkowski S. First passage times as environmental safety indicators: carboxyhemoglobin from cigarette smoke. *Biometrics 1979; 35:* 539–548

36   Wright GR, Shephard RJ. Physiological effects of carbon monoxide. *Int Rev Physiol 1979; 20:* 311–368

Chapter Three

SMOKING AND DISEASES OF THE LUNG

CANCER OF THE LUNG

No advances have occurred in the treatment of lung cancer in recent years that shift the emphasis in the control of this disease away from prevention. Likewise no developments in our understanding of the causation of lung cancer have shifted emphasis away from cigarette smoking as the chief culprit. Limited progress has been made in determining why some subjects are unduly susceptible to the carcinogenic effects of cigarette smoke, though no categories of regular cigarette smokers can be identified who are safe from the disease (see Chapter 5).

There have been important trends in lung cancer mortality in the last decade. In the United Kingdom death rates from lung cancer in men have declined in recent years, a trend already becoming evident in those in early middle age at the time of the publication of the last Royal College of Physicians report [1]. During the 1950s annual mortality for lung cancer in middle-aged men levelled off and by the 1960s had begun to fall. A few years later a similar phenomenon occurred in older men and lung cancer mortality is now rising only in the very oldest age groups of men in this country (Figure 3.1). In the United States [2] death rates in men have continued to rise in most age groups except in the very youngest, where there is a slight downward trend. In contrast to the trends in men, lung cancer mortality continues to rise steeply in women in both countries, emphasising that they are probably as susceptible to the carcinogenic effects of cigarette smoke as are men. By the early 1980s lung cancer mortality for women in the United States is likely to exceed that of breast cancer, and, unless large changes in female smoking habits occur, these increases are likely to continue for at least the remainder of this century. The one encouraging trend is a decline in the rate of lung cancer in women in the younger age groups in the United Kingdom (Figure 3.1), even though the small numbers involved make only a trivial contribution to the total deaths.

The key to understanding these trends in national lung cancer statistics lies in an appreciation of the influence of cigarette usage throughout adult life on mortality in middle and old age. Changes in current mortality relate to patterns of smoking several decades before, as well as current smoking habits. Thus, the current increase in United States male and female lung cancer mortality in late middle age are likely to be due to the delayed effects of increases in cigarette consumption by young United States adults 30 or more years ago. Likewise

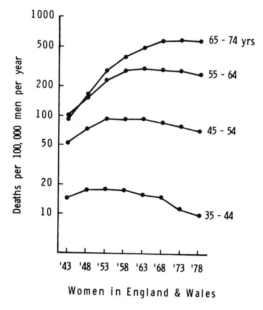

Figure 3.1. Lung cancer deaths in men and women in England and Wales. Death rates per 100,000 per year between 1943 and 1978 are shown for four age groups each covering a span of 10 years. The decline in mortality seen in all except the oldest men is only just becoming evident in the youngest women

the current increases in United Kingdom female lung cancer deaths may chiefly reflect the delayed effects of increases in cigarette usage by young British women during, or even before, World War II. The trends in male lung cancer deaths in the United Kingdom do not follow this pattern and so are of particular interest.

Britain is unusual among developed countries in being one of the first where young men adopted cigarette smoking on a wide scale. After a steady rise throughout World War II, male cigarette consumption then dropped temporarily before settling out at an approximately constant level for the next 25 to 30 years (see Figure 1.1). Because of this, studies in British men offer unusual opportunities for evaluating the effects of changing smoking habits. Once the relatively constant cigarette consumption of British men had rendered lung cancer mortality constant, it became possible to assess the significance for health of changing the content in cigarettes of various harmful or potentially harmful constituents. Thus there are good reasons to suppose that the recent welcome downward trend in British male lung cancer mortality may be related to reductions in the tar and nicotine content of cigarettes.

TABLE 3.1. Changes in England and Wales male lung cancer death rates in early middle age since tar deliveries have been reduced

Age at time of observation	Death rates per million men from cancers of the respiratory tract, excluding larynx		Ratio
	Men born in about 1910, and observed in 1940–1960	Men born in about 1930–1950, and observed in 1980	
30–34	39**	13	0.3
35–39	98**	45	0.5
40–44	253**	134	0.5
45–49	597**	378*	0.6

* High mean tar intake only in first decade or so of smoking history

** High mean tar intake throughout smoking history

Table 3.1 illustrates the type of data on which this conclusion is based. Death rates from lung cancer are listed for men born in 1910, who would have smoked cigarettes with high tar yield throughout their smoking history. These are contrasted with rates taken in 1980 for men born 20 to 40 years later, most of whom would have smoked cigarettes with rapidly decreasing tar yields for up to 20 years (see Figure 9.1 for changes in yields). To take as an example those men observed at 40 to 48 years of age, death rates for the second group of men are seen to be half those of the first. It is important to note that mean cigarette consumption for men aged 30 to 50 had not changed greatly in the two decades before 1980, and that trends have not been influenced by changes in the curative treatment of lung cancer. In Finland, where male cigarette smoking also began so long ago that the trends had nearly flattened out by the 1950s, male lung cancer rates in early middle age have likewise been approximately halved over the past 20 years [2]. The wider implications of such findings in relation to the development of less dangerous cigarettes are taken up in Chapter 9.

The influence of duration of smoking on lung cancer risk has been emphasised in recent years. A specific illustration (Figure 3.2) of this

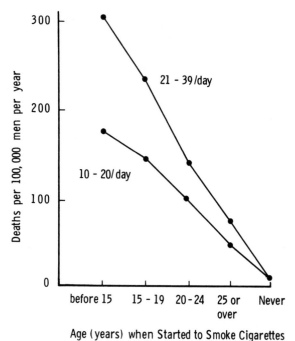

Figure 3.2. Lung cancer in male US Veterans as rates per 100,000 men per year and analysed for two consumption rates (10–20 and 21–39 cigarettes per day) according to age when the subject started smoking. The younger the age at which smoking was started, the higher was the risk of lung cancer

effect comes from lung cancer mortality rates in current smokers of cigarettes amongst US Veterans [3]. Analysis of the data underlines the importance of exposure to cigarette smoke early in life. Lung cancer risk at the age of 60 is three times as great in those starting to smoke at around the age of 15 as it is in those who do not start smoking for a further 10 years. Thus current patterns of lung cancer in the elderly are strongly influenced by the smoking habits of teenagers 40 or 50 years earlier.

Emphasis on the effects of smoking habits in early adult life is not to deny the influence on lung cancer risk of recent smoking habits. The beneficial effects of stopping smoking illustrate this [4]. Proper interpretation again relies on an understanding of the influence of duration of smoking. Reference to Table 3.2 shows that the annual

TABLE 3.2. Approximate* effects of various durations of cigarette smoking on annual incidence of lung cancer

Years of cigarette smoking	Annual excess incidence	
	Moderate smokers	Heavy smokers
15	0.005%	0.01%
30	0.1%	0.2%
45	0.5%	1%
(60)	(1.5%?)	(3%?)

* Estimated from data reported by Doll and Peto [4] for male British doctors. The cumulative risks would be far greater than these annual risks, of course, so an eventual total of over 10 per cent of regular cigarette smokers may die of tobacco-induced cancer, depending on the number and type of cigarettes smoked

excess risk of lung cancer amongst British male doctors after 30 years of moderate smoking was about one in a thousand (0.1%). If smoking is stopped at this stage the annual excess incidence remains roughly constant thereafter. If smoking is continued, however, it is seen that the excess risk rises after a further 15 years to five in a thousand. Thus stopping smoking after 30 years reduces the risk of developing lung cancer 15 years later by about 80 per cent. Similar results hold for heavy smokers. This does *not* imply that the absolute risk of lung cancer disappears: ex-smokers can still develop lung cancer and the chief determinant of their increased risk is the total duration of their smoking earlier in life. It does, however, imply that if smokers give up before they have developed cancer as a result of their habit, then they are likely to avoid most of the subsequent risk of this disease that they would otherwise incur.

CHRONIC LUNG DISEASE

The classification of those chronic lung diseases that are due to smoking has been simplified during the past few years by the realisation that, lung cancer apart, the adverse effects of cigarette smoke on the lungs may be separated into two quite distinct conditions.

On the one hand there is *chronic mucus hypersecretion*, which causes persistent cough with phlegm and fits with the original definition of simple chronic bronchitis. This condition arises chiefly in the large airways, usually clears up when the subject stops smoking and does not on its own carry any substantial risk of death.

On the other hand there is *chronic obstructive lung disease**, which causes difficulty in breathing due to narrowing of the air passages in the lungs. This condition originates chiefly in the small airways, includes a variable element of destruction of peripheral lung units, is progressive and largely irreversible and may ultimately lead to disability and death.

Although both conditions may be produced by smoking and can co-exist in a given individual, they are distinct, not least in that the obstructive condition is responsible for much disability and death, whereas the mucus hypersecretion does not of itself influence life expectancy. Patients with either condition do, however, share a strong tendency to suffer from acute infective illnesses for which the term 'bronchitis', implying as it does infection in the bronchial tree, is frequently used and not inappropriate. These infective illnesses are substantial causes of discomfort and of absence from work through sickness. Airways obstruction is often more severe during an infective episode but recovery is usual, and these episodes do not seem to accelerate the progression of chronic obstructive lung disease [5].

The obstructive syndrome is as specifically related to smoking as is lung cancer, and in one prospective survey of the effects of smoking on mortality (that among British doctors) the relative risk for chronic obstructive lung disease was even more extreme than that for lung cancer [4]. Despite this, in discussing the health effects of tobacco, there has generally been far more emphasis on lung cancer than on this more disabling, but equally fatal disorder.

The onset of the disease is perhaps best characterised by patterns of change in the lung function test known as the one-second forced expiratory volume (FEV_1).** These are outlined in Figure 3.3 [5] where for simplicity FEV_1 is expressed as a percentage of what it would have been at age 25. FEV_1 loss is typically a slow process, spread out over several decades, rather than a sudden change from normality to disease. Moreover, it tends to be largely irreversible and once FEV_1 falls to about one litre the subject is usually disabled. Among non-smokers the normal range of rates of loss of FEV_1 is

---

*   Equivalent terms are: chronic airflow obstruction, chronic obstructive pulmonary disease chronic non-specific lung disease. The composite term chronic bronchitis and emphysema is also still used, but the extent to which chronic obstructive lung disease is due to emphysema, destruction of lung units, is quite variable and not readily determinable in life.

** FEV_1 is defined as the maximal amount of air that can be expelled during the first second of forced expiration after a full deep breath in. Its value should be standardised for age, sex and height (e.g. by dividing FEV_1 by the square or the cube of height).

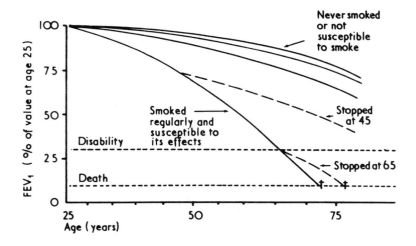

Figure 3.3. Diagrammatic representation of decline in lung function with age based on actual data [5] and represented by percentage of one-second forced expiratory volume at age 25 in various population groups. The regular smoker who is susceptible to the damaging effects of cigarette smoke on the airways will show a rapid decline in function, though this can be slowed by stopping smoking

narrow and almost all non-smokers reach the age at which they die from another cause long before becoming disabled by obstructed airways. Among smokers, however, the range of rates of loss of FEV_1 is much wider. For reasons that are still obscure, some smokers do not suffer a particularly rapid rate of loss of FEV_1 as a result of their smoking. By contrast, some 'susceptible' smokers suffer such unusually rapid rates of loss of FEV_1 that if they continue to smoke they will be first disabled and then killed by their obstructive lung disease. Among these 'susceptible' smokers the effects of stopping smoking are of critical importance. If such people stop smoking their FEV_1 will not recover, but their subsequent rate of loss of FEV_1 will usually revert to about that seen in non-smokers (Figure 3.3). Thus if susceptible smokers stop well before they are disabled, they will not die from chronic obstructive lung disease, but if they do not stop until they are disabled, then they are likely to die from it within a few years. Indeed, because progressive respiratory disability may cause people to stop smoking, deaths from this disease tend to occur not in continuing smokers but among people whose disease has led them to stop smoking a few years previously [4].

It would be of considerable help in picking out the susceptible smoker if the condition could be diagnosed in its early stages long before the FEV_1 has become clearly abnormal. Regrettably, unequivocal changes on the chest radiograph are not evident until late in the disease [6], and none of the various tests of lung function thus far devised has been proved to predict reliably early in life which smokers will develop severe chronic obstructive lung disease in their later years [7].

Although for people in their twenties and thirties lung function tests may not clearly indicate which smokers are heading for serious trouble, by middle age the simple FEV_1 is remarkably informative.

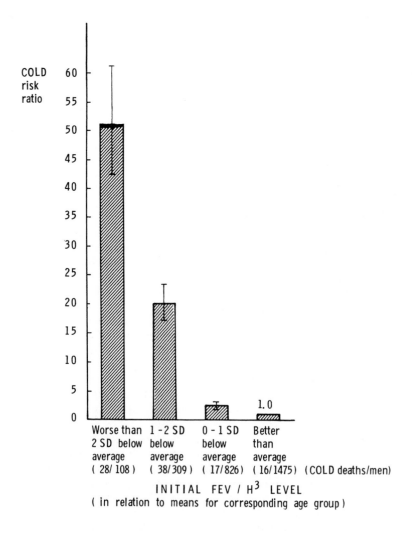

Figure 3.4. Histogram to illustrate the strikingly high risk of the subsequent development of chronic obstructive lung disease (COLD) for men who already have lung function significantly below average in early middle life [8]

Various surveys of British men carried out in the 1950s and early 1960s are just now yielding sufficient data on deaths from chronic obstructive lung disease to draw conclusions on this point [8]. The single original FEV_1 (measured when these men were in their fifties) has been used to predict reliably which men would have a high risk of death from chronic obstructive lung disease during the subsequent twenty-odd years (Figure 3.4). By contrast, among men of similar age and FEV_1, the presence or absence of chronic mucus hypersecretion (or a recent history of chest infections) was not significantly related to subsequent mortality from chronic obstructive lung disease.

As with all the main tobacco-related diseases, however, the chief problem is no longer .whether tobacco causes the disease or not, but rather what can be done to avoid these effects of tobacco. The best way is to cease smoking, and the next to reduce the amount smoked. The age-standardised chronic obstructive lung disease death rates per 100,000 British doctors who smoked 0, 1−14, 15−24 and 25+ cigarettes a day were 3, 51, 78 and 114 respectively [4], which suggests that diminution of the dose does produce diminution of the effect.

A parallel strategy that may be effective is to encourage the continued development and use of less hazardous cigarettes. Unfortunately, for chronic obstructive disease even more than for lung cancer, it is difficult to determine directly what constitutes a less hazardous cigarette. There are two main reasons for this.

The first is that it is still not known how cigarette smoking causes chronic obstructive lung disease. The main suggestions, which were reviewed in the US Surgeon-General's (1979) report on Smoking and Health [9], are interference with the clearance of mucus from the airways, interference with the lung's defence against infection and, perhaps more promising, interference with the balance of enzymes which maintain the structural integrity of the lungs (for further details see Chapter 5). Whilst this uncertainty remains, the hazards of different types of cigarette must be determined by direct epidemiological observation.

Unfortunately, the second source of difficulty is epidemiological. It arises because chronic obstructive lung disease is the end result of a gradual loss of FEV_1 over many decades, and cigarette usage has changed so fast that current patterns of use may bear little relation to usage 20 or 30 years ago. Moreover, just as low FEV_1 causes people to stop or diminish their smoking, so may it also encourage them to switch to a low tar brand. If this is so, standard epidemiological studies of the smoking habits of people disabled by low FEV_1 might even misleadingly suggest that switching to low tar cigarettes and/or stopping smoking were peculiarly hazardous.

Despite these problems there is some epidemiological evidence that lower tar cigarettes are preferable, and this is considered in Chapter 9.

Other causes of chronic obstructive lung disease

Two observations indicate that some extrinsic factors must exist that alone or in conjunction with smoking are responsible for some of the mortality due to chronic obstructive lung disease. The first is that there was no dramatic rise in death rates from chronic obstructive lung disease that paralleled the rise in tobacco consumption as described earlier for lung cancer mortality (Figure 3.1). Secondly, there are striking differences between social classes I and V in chronic obstructive lung disease death certification that cannot be explained in terms of differences in smoking habits alone (Table 3.3). Air pollution, which

TABLE 3.3. Mortality from chronic obstructive lung disease: male and female social class gradients in 1961. Social class was an important correlate of chronic obstructive lung disease death certification rates at a time when smoking habits were fairly similar in all social classes

| Social class | 'Bronchitis' (chiefly COLD*): Standardised mortality ratios in 1961 among people aged 15–64 | |
	Males by own occupation	Married females, by husband's occupation
I	28	33
II	50	51
III	97	102
IV	116	118
V	194	196

* 7th ICD 500–502:

COLD = chronic obstructive lung disease

has certainly decreased, and might be more important in working class families, may modify the effects of tobacco. Unfortunately, no proper studies exist of the separate and joint effects of tobacco and air pollution in childhood or adult life on chronic obstructive lung disease, though air pollution has been shown to increase mucus hypersecretion [10]. Other factors that may influence susceptibility are discussed in Chapter 5, but whilst such factors undoubtedly exist it must be emphasised that at present only the effects of tobacco are reliably known to be of substantial importance.

References

1   Office of Population Censuses and Surveys. *Trends in Respiratory Mortality 1981; Series DH1, No. 7.* London: HMSO

2   Doll R, Peto R. Trends in lung cancer death rates in relation to cigarette usage and tar yields. Appendix E in: The Causes of Cancer. *J Natl Cancer Inst 1981; 66:* 1191–1308

3   Kahn HA. The Dorn study of smoking and mortality among US veterans: a report on eight and one half years of observation. In Haenszel W, ed. *Natl Cancer Inst Monogr 19; 1966:* 1–125

4   Doll R, Peto R. Mortality in relation to smoking: 20 years' observations on male British doctors. *Br Med J 1976; 4:* 1525–1536

5   Fletcher CM, Peto R. The natural history of chronic airflow obstruction. *Br Med J 1977; 1:* 1645–1648

6   Musk AW. Validation of the plain chest radiograph for epidemiologic studies of airflow obstruction. *Am J Epidemiol 1982; 116:* 801–807

7   Tattersall SF, Benson MK, Hunter D et al. The use of tests of peripheral lung function for predicting future disability from airflow obstruction in middle-aged smokers. *Am Rev Respir Dis 1978; 118:* 1035–1050

8   Peto R, Speizer FE, Cochrane AL et al. The relevance in adults of airflow obstruction, but not of mucus hypersecretion, to mortality from chronic lung disease: 20-year results from prospective surveys. *Am Rev Respir Dis 1983:* in press

9   US Surgeon-General. *Smoking and Health: A Report of the Surgeon-General.* DHEW Publication No PHS 79-50066. Washington DC: US Government Printing Office. 1979

10   Lambert PM, Reid DD. Smoking, air pollution, and bronchitis in Britain. *Lancet 1970; i:* 853–857

Chapter Four

SMOKING AND DISEASES OF THE HEART AND BLOOD VESSELS

HEART DISEASE

Although public concern has continued to focus on the danger of lung cancer, diseases of the heart and blood vessels still account for over one-third of all the excess deaths in smokers. Coronary heart disease, leading to death by myocardial infarction, is the major problem. Though the relative risk of developing coronary heart disease is much less than that for lung cancer or chronic bronchitis, because the disease is more common, the number of heart disease deaths attributable to smoking is greater than for either of these lung disorders.

This effect was clearly illustrated in the British doctors study [1] (Table 4.1). Men under 65 years of age smoking 25 or more cigarettes

TABLE 4.1. Deaths per 100,000 men per year from coronary heart disease in British male doctors [1]

| Age | Annual death rate per 100,000 men | | | | Relative mortality risk of smoking 25+ cigarettes/day |
| | Non-smokers | Smokers: cigarettes per day | | | |
		1–14	15–24	25+	
45	7	46	61	104	14.8
45–54	118	220	368	393	3.3
55–64	531	742	819	1,025	1.9
65	166	278	358	427	2.6

a day had a relative risk of developing coronary heart disease of 2.6 times that of non-smokers, and older men had very little increased risk. However, overall in the study, 3,191 of these male doctors died of coronary heart disease compared with only 441 dying from lung cancer. So even though only about 30 per cent of the heart disease deaths are attributable to smoking, the actual number of excess deaths attributable to smoking is much greater than for lung cancer. Deaths from coronary heart disease in men in England and Wales during 1980 represented 31 per cent of all deaths, this figure being more than three times the number of deaths due to lung cancer; in women in the same year nearly eight times as many died from coronary heart disease as from lung cancer [2].

A second feature which emerges in epidemiological surveys which have examined the relation between smoking and coronary heart disease is the age effect. Table 4.1 shows that the relative risk of coronary heart disease in smokers falls from 14.8 in those under 45 years, to 1.9 in those 55–64 years. Similar trends appear in major American studies. The prospective study of one million persons by the American Cancer Society [3] showed, for example, that men smoking 20–39 cigarettes a day had a relative risk of coronary heart disease 3.76 times that of non-smokers aged 40–49, this figure falling to 1.49 for those aged 70–79. The more recent Pooling Project [4] combined results from eight American studies totalling 6,975 men aged 40–59 years and again confirmed the trend (four to five times relative risk in the youngest men down to 1.7 times in older men). It is important to emphasise that, despite this, it is among older people that the majority of the excess deaths due to smoking occur. The reasons for the decline in the relative importance of cigarette smoking with age are not totally clear, but one likely explanation is that the most susceptible smokers have already been killed by their coronary heart disease in early middle life.

The Pooling Project illustrated, as had previous surveys, the dose response relationship between the number of cigarettes smoked and relative risk (Table 4.2). Concerning pipe and cigar smokers the Pooling

TABLE 4.2

Smoking category	Relative risk
Non-smoker	1.0
Ex-smoker	1.2
Pipe/cigars only	1.3
Cigarettes <½ pack/day	1.0
½ pack/day	1.9
1 pack/day	2.2
>1 pack/day	3.4

Project report commented: "Their position on the continuum of risk is not entirely clear. Risk is definitely below that of men who smoke a pack or more of cigarettes . . . . It has not been established that the risk of pipe and cigar smokers is greater than that of the low group (i.e. those smoking less than 10 cigarettes a day)". On the other hand in a follow-up study of 5,249 Copenhagen men aged 40 to 57 there were 1,208 regular smokers of cheroots [5]. Their risk of developing myocardial infarction was 2.8 times that of non-smokers (4.2 for those smoking more than six daily).

The relationship between cigarette consumption and relative risk of coronary heart disease appears to be independent of other factors such as raised serum cholesterol [6], hypertension [7], obesity [8], physical inactivity [9], personality type and electrocardiographic changes [10]. Nevertheless, there is no doubt that the causation of coronary heart disease is multi-factorial. Smoking is one of three major risk factors, raised blood pressure and the concentration of blood cholesterol being the other two. The Pooling Project can be used to illustrate this. Like smoking, each of the other two factors increases the risk of coronary heart disease by about two-and-a-half-fold. If a subject is above average for all three factors the risk becomes eight times greater than for those who have below average figures for each of the three risk factors.

The influence of multiple factors is evident in national statistics for coronary heart disease. Striking differences exist between countries. Finland and Northern Ireland headed the table (in 1977) at more than 700 deaths per 100,000 men aged 35–74 each year. Southern European countries had rates around 200 per 100,000 and Japan was at the bottom of the list with 88 per 100,000 [11]. Important movement has occurred within this league table, particularly a decline in United States figures over the 1950s and 1960s. Rates have also fallen in Australia, Belgium and a few other countries. In the United Kingdom rates have certainly reached a plateau but there are as yet only the slightest hints of a downward trend [12,13].

Recent studies of ex-smokers support the earlier view that most of the association between cigarette smoking and coronary heart disease is causal. In Finland, of 648 men who survived one year after myocardial infarction, it was found that deaths (age-adjusted) in the next four years were 2.3 times greater for continuing smokers than for non-smokers [14]. In those who stopped smoking after the attack the risk was almost identical with that of non-smokers. In the Framingham survey those who stopped smoking after a heart attack had a death rate six years later that was 62 per cent less than that of those who continued smoking [15], despite the fact that both smokers and non-smokers still continued to have an equal number of non-fatal heart attacks. Furthermore, the beneficial effects of stopping smoking persist for at least 15 years after a myocardial infarction [16]. Thus, though the damage to the coronary arteries that predisposes to a heart attack probably takes years to accumulate, it is important to realise how quickly the excess risk diminishes in those who give up smoking after an attack and for how long the benefit lasts. This strongly suggests that smoking acts in some important way in determining the fatal event in coronary heart disease, and therefore stopping smoking is the single most important action that can be taken in preventing the thousands of deaths due to this condition.

It is unfortunate that not all those who are given smoking advice do in fact stop smoking. In a randomised controlled trial of the effects of smoking cessation in middle-aged civil servants, Rose and co-workers [17] reported that 10-year coronary heart disease mortality was only 18 per cent lower in those receiving advice as compared with controls, a difference not statistically significant.

This section has concentrated on evidence referring to men. Smoking is equally important in the causation of coronary heart disease in women and this is discussed more fully in Chapter 7.

By what mechanisms does smoking cause coronary heart disease?

A necropsy study from Boston, USA [18] has confirmed the finding of more advanced narrowing of coronary arteries in smokers, particularly heavy smokers. In addition, there was a new finding, namely severe thickening of the smallest arteries supplying the heart. This occurred in 91 per cent of those who had smoked 40 or more cigarettes daily, in 48 per cent of those smoking less than 20 cigarettes daily and in none of those who had never smoked regularly.

A survey of men and women industrial workers in north-west London has shown that the ability of the blood to dissolve blood clots was significantly reduced in smokers, although the effect was not large [19].

It seems that smoking may promote the formation of fatty plaques on the surface of blood vessels, cause thickening of the small vessels of the heart and encourage blood clots, as well as reduce the heart's oxygen supply and make it more irritable so that it does not beat regularly. Any or all of these mechanisms could contribute to death from heart disease, but exactly how this is brought about is not known.

What constituents of smoke are responsible?

A report from the Tobacco Research Council [20] that smokers of filter cigarettes had a 25 per cent reduction in coronary heart disease deaths has not been confirmed either in Britain [21] or in the United States [22]. The latter report is a further study of the whole population of Framingham. This found that smokers of filter cigarettes suffered as many heart attacks as did smokers of non-filter cigarettes. This would imply that the harmful constituents are in the gases which get through the filters. Most attention is focused on nicotine and carbon monoxide. Though nicotine certainly has adverse effects on the heart and blood vessels (Chapter 2), Wald's group [23] has adduced a further argument against the role of nicotine as a cardiac risk factor. They found that urinary cotinine levels (taken as a marker for nicotine retention) are no higher in cigarette smokers, who have a high risk of coronary heart disease, than in pipe smokers, who have a low risk. Pipe smokers do, however, have low levels of blood carbon monoxide.

Carbon monoxide binds to the pigment in red blood cells, haemoglobin, which normally transports oxygen from the lungs to the tissues. The pigment compound carboxyhaemoglobin is formed, leaving less haemoglobin to carry oxygen. Hence, when more than half of the haemoglobin is converted to carboxyhaemoglobin, as occurs with coal gas poisoning, death usually results from lack of oxygen in the brain and heart.

Habitual cigarette smokers usually have between three and seven per cent of their haemoglobin converted to carboxyhaemoglobin [24].

Although it is arguably harmful for up to seven per cent of the oxygen-carrying capacity of the blood to be rendered ineffective, there is some controversy as to the precise health consequences of this. In people healthy in other respects no harm seems to follow [25]. Habitual smokers, however, show an increase in the total number of red blood cells, which appears to represent a compensation for the presence of the carboxyhaemoglobin [26]. This may itself be harmful since it makes the blood thicker and more likely to clot. Undoubtedly in smokers whose circulation is already compromised, even a modest decrease in blood oxygen-carrying capacity can have adverse effects. In patients with angina or other evidence of insufficiency of the coronary arteries, even exposure to a minor amount of carbon monoxide has been shown to decrease effort tolerance and make the angina worse [27].

Evidence against carbon monoxide from epidemiological studies remains weak: it could be simply a marker for some other inhalant. The last College report described how Wald and others [28] found that blood carbon monoxide concentrations were good predictors of coronary heart disease risk. In a later Finnish cross-sectional study [29] blood carbon monoxide did not show any stronger relation to prevalence of atherosclerotic disease than did a simple smoking history. This discrepancy may reflect only the varying reliability of the smoking history.

A recent survey in Boston, analysing the risk of a first (non-fatal) myocardial infarction in men under 55 years of age, found that risk was unrelated to either the nicotine or the carbon monoxide yield of the cigarettes they had been smoking [30]. This study and several others of similar type did not assess inhaling habits. Measured yields are those determined using smoking machines, and it is possible that smoking behaviour has an important influence on the delivery of nicotine and carbon monoxide to the smoker. The 10-year mortality study of British civil servants found that coronary heart disease risk was greater among smokers who said that they inhaled [31]. It was also related to tar/nicotine yield, but only among the 'inhalers' — the reverse of what was found for lung cancer. The authors concluded: "It appears that there are subtle interactions between the amount smoked, the tar/nicotine yield of the cigarette, and the style of smoking. Thus the effects of a change in cigarette characteristics are hard to predict, and they may be different for respiratory and cardiovascular disease."

In summary, we still do not know what constituent of cigarette smoke is responsible for the cardiovascular risk, which is nevertheless the main cause of the excess mortality of smokers. It might be carbon monoxide, and the mere possibility justifies attempts to reduce the carbon monoxide yield of cigarettes. Whatever the responsible factor or factors may be, their retention in the lungs and circulating blood and the consequent damage to the heart are enhanced by inhalation, so that anything which tends to increase inhalation is likely to increase the cardiovascular risk and hence could increase the overall mortality risk.

These considerations led the recent WHO Expert Committee on the Prevention of Coronary Heart Disease [32] to conclude: "As far as coronary heart disease is concerned, present evidence does not support promotion of the so-called 'safer cigarette', i.e. one of low tar/nicotine yields."

Disease of the peripheral circulation

Atherosclerosis of the peripheral arteries supplying the lower limbs causes leg pain on walking (intermittent claudication), pain in the feet at rest or even tissue death or gangrene. Similar disease which narrows the carotid arteries supplying the brain may cause strokes. Occasionally an arteriosclerotic artery in any part of the body can dilate to form an aneurysm, which may burst causing fatal haemorrhage. More than 90 per cent of patients suffering from any of these diseases have smoked at least 20 cigarettes a day for 20 years or more. Very few are lifelong non-smokers [33].

If patients with intermittent claudication continue to smoke, rest pain or gangrene leading to amputation is more likely to occur, and symptoms are more likely to develop in previously asymptomatic limbs [34]. In an attempt to avoid this plight arterial reconstruction or by-pass surgery is frequently performed. Regrettably these grafts sometimes fail because they become blocked by clots. Two studies report a high incidence of by-pass failure among those patients who continued to smoke after surgery, compared with those who did not [35,36]. Grafts in patients who continued to smoke more than five cigarettes per day were three to four times more likely to fail than those in patients who smoked less, even though there was no correlation between pre-operative smoking habits and the immediate outcome of the operation [37].

Smokers cannot be relied upon to report their smoking habits accurately [38]. Confirmation of continued smoking can be obtained with carboxyhaemoglobin [39] or thiocyanate [40] levels in the blood. Carboxyhaemoglobin levels have been found to be significantly higher in patients whose arterial reconstructions failed within five years, than in those in whom the grafts were successful [41]. Assessments of the blood supply to the legs in terms of resting ankle blood pressure and exercise ability revealed continued deterioration in patients who continued to smoke compared with improvement in those who stopped smoking [42]. Smoking has also been shown to be a factor leading to failure by thrombosis of artery to vein shunts constructed to facilitate haemodialysis in patients with kidney failure [43].

Conclusions

There is little doubt about the importance of smoking in relation to diseases of the heart and blood vessels. Whilst mechanisms are still imperfectly understood, the basic clinical facts stand firm. Coronary heart disease is the major killer among the smoking-related diseases, and the rewards for stopping are both immediate and substantial. Amputation due to vascular disease in the legs is a tragic complication of smoking and for those whose legs are saved by arterial reconstruction, continued smoking can undo all the benefit gained.

References

1   Doll R, Peto R. Mortality in relation to smoking: 20 years' observations on male British doctors. *Br Med J 1976; 4:* 1525–1536
2   UK Mortality Statistics. London: HMSO. 1981
3   Hammond EC. Smoking in relation to the death rates of one million men and women. In Haenszel W, ed. *Natl Cancer Inst Monogr 19 1966:* 127–204
4   The Pooling Project Research Group. Relationship of blood pressure, serum cholesterol, smoking habit, relative weight and ECG abnormalities to incidence of major coronary events: final report of the Pooling Project. *J Chronic Dis 1978; 31:* 201–306
5   Gyntelberg F, Lauridsen L, Pedersen PB, Schubell K. Smoking and risk of myocardial infarction in Copenhagen men aged 40–59 with special reference to cheroot smoking. *Lancet 1981; i:* 987–989
6   Stamler J, Berkson DM, Levinson M et al. Coronary artery disease. Status of preventive efforts. *Arch Environ Health 1966; 13:* 322–335
7   Borhani NO, Hechter HH, Breslow L. Report of a 10-year follow-up study of the San Francisco longshoremen. Mortality from coronary heart disease and from all causes. *J Chronic Dis 1963; 16:* 1251–1266
8   Berkson DM et al. An important risk factor for coronary mortality – ten-year experience of The People's Gas Co epidemiologic study (1958–68). In Jones RJ, ed. *Atherosclerosis. Proceedings of the Second International Symposium.* New York: Springer-Verlag. 1970: 382–389
9   Shapiro S, Weinblatt E, Frank CW, Sager RV. Incidence of coronary heart disease in a population insured for medical care (HIP). Myocardial infarction. *Am J Public Health 1969; 59:* Suppl 2: 1–101
10   Keys A. *A Multivariate Analysis of Health and Coronary Heart Disease in Seven Countries.* Cambridge, Massachusetts: Harvard University Press. 1980
11   WHO Annual Statistics for Coronary Heart Disease Mortality. Geneva: World Health Organization
12   Heller RF, Hayward D, Hobbs MST. Decline in rate of death from ischaemic heart disease in the United Kingdom. *Br Med J 1983; 286:* 260–262
13   Tunstall-Pedoe D, Kenicer M, Iannoukos L. Decline in rate of death from ischaemic heart disease in the United Kingdom. *Br Med J 1983; 286:* 560
14   Pohjola S. Siltanen P, Romo M. Five-year survival of 728 patients after myocardial infarction. *Br Heart J 1980; 43:* 176–183
15   Sparrow D, Dawber TR, Colton T. The influence of cigarette smoking on prognosis after a first myocardial infarction. *J Chronic Dis 1978;31:*425–432
16   Daly LE, Mulcahy R, Graham IM, Hickey N. Long-term effect on mortality of stopping smoking after unstable angina and myocardial infarction. *Br Med J 1983; 287:* 324–326
17   Rose G, Hamilton PJS, Colwell L, Shipley M. A randomised controlled trial of anti-smoking advice: 10-year results. *J Epidemiol Community Health 1982; 36:* 102–108

18   Auerbach O, Carter HW, Garfinkel L, Hammond EC. Cigarette smoking and coronary heart disease, a macroscopic and microscopic study. *Chest 1976; 70:* 697–705

19   Meade TW, Chakrabarti R, Haines AP et al. Characteristics affecting fibrinolytic activity and plasma fibrinogen concentrations. *Br Med J 1979; 1:* 143–156

20   Dean G, Lee PN, Todd GF, Wilken AJ. *Report on a Second Retrospective Mortality Study in North-east England. 1. Factors Related to Mortality from Lung Cancer, Bronchitis, Heart Disease and Stroke in Cleveland County, with Particular Emphasis on the Relative Risks Associated with Smoking Filter and Plain Cigarettes. Research Paper 14.* London: Tobacco Research Council. 1977

21   Hawthorne VM, Fry JS. Smoking and health: the association between smoking behaviour, total mortality, and cardiorespiratory disease in west central Scotland. *J Epidemiol Community Health 1978; 32:* 260–266

22   Castelli WP, Garrison RJ, Dawber TR et al. The filter cigarette and coronary heart disease: the Framingham study. *Lancet 1981; ii:* 109–113

23   Wald NJ, Idle M, Boreham J et al. Serum cotinine levels in pipe smokers: evidence against nicotine as cause of coronary heart disease. *Lancet 1981; ii:* 775–777

24   Cohen SI, Perkins NM, Ury HK, Goldsmith JH. Carbon monoxide uptake in cigarette smoking. *Arch Environ Health 1971; 22:* 55–60

25   Mikulka P, O'Donnell R, Hernig P, Theodore J. The effect of carbon monoxide on human performance. *Ann NY Acad Sci 1970; 174:* 409–420

26   Eisen ME, Hammond EC. The effect of smoking on packed cell volume, red cell counts, haemoglobin and platelet counts. *J Can Med Assoc 1956; 75:* 520–527

27   Ayres SM, Gianelli S, Muller H. Myocardial and systemic responses to carboxy haemoglobin. *Ann NY Acad Sci 1970; 174:* 268–293

28   Wald N, Howard S, Smith PG, Kjeldsen K. Association between atherosclerotic diseases and carboxyhaemoglobin levels in tobacco smokers. *Br Med J 1973; 1:* 761–765

29   Heliövaara M, Karvonen MJ, Vilhunen R, Punsar S. Smoking, carbon monoxide, and atherosclerotic diseases. *Br Med J 1978; 1:* 268–270

30   Kaufman DW, Helmrich SP, Rosenberg L et al. Nicotine and carbon monoxide content of cigarette smoke and the risk of myocardial infarction in young men. *N Engl J Med 1983; 308:* 409–413

31   Higgenbottam T, Shipley MJ, Rose G. Cigarettes, lung cancer and coronary heart disease: the effects of inhalation and tar yield. *J Epidemiol Community Health 1982; 36:* 113–117

32   World Health Organization. *The Prevention of Coronary Heart Disease: Report of an Expert Committee.* Geneva: World Health Organization. 1982

33   Laing SP, Greenhalgh RM, Taylor GW. The prevalence of cigarette smoking in patients with peripheral arterial disease. In Greenhalgh RM, ed. *Smoking and Arterial Disease.* London: Pitman Medical. 1981

34   Hughson WG, Mann JI, Tibbs DJ et al. Intermittent claudication: factors determining outcome. *Br Med J 1978; 1:* 1377–1379

35   Wray R, DePalma RC, Hubay CH. Late occlusion of aorto-femoral bypass grafts; influence of cigarette smoking. *Surgery 1971; 70:* 969–973

36   Robicsek F, Dougherty HK, Mullen DC et al. The effect of continued cigarette smoking on the patency of synthetic grafts in Leriche Syndrome. *J Thorac Cardiovasc Surg 1975; 70:* 107–113

37   Myers KA, King RB, Scott DF et al. The effect of smoking on the later patency of arterial reconstructions in the legs. *Br J Surg 1978; 65:* 267–271

38   Sillett RW, Wilson MB, Malcolm RE, Ball KP. Deception among smokers. *Br Med J 1978; 2:* 1185–1186

39   Castelden CM, Cole PV. Variations in carboxyhaemoglobin levels in smokers. *Br Med J 1974; 4:* 736–738

40   Vesey CJ, Saloojee Y, Cole PV, Russell MAH. Blood carboxyhaemoglobin, plasma thiocyanate and cigarette consumption: implications for epidemiological studies in smokers. *Br Med J 1982; 284:* 1516–1518

41   Greenhalgh RM, Laing SP, Cole PV, Taylor GW. Smoking and arterial reconstruction. *Br J Surg 1981; 68:* 605–607

42   Quick CRG, Cotton LT. The measured effect of stopping smoking on intermittent claudication. *Br J Surg 1982; 69:* Suppl June: 24–26

43   Griffin PJA, Davies F, Salaman JR, Coles GA. Effects of smoking on long term patency of arterio-venous fistulae. *Br Med J 1983; 286:* 685–686

Chapter Five

SUSCEPTIBILITY TO THE SMOKING HAZARD

INTRODUCTION

The Director of the National Cancer Institute National Cancer Programme wrote in 1977: "Scientists still are unable to explain . . . . why some heavy smokers apparently are resistant to the development of lung cancer . . .". Some smokers also appear to survive the onslaught of coronary heart disease and of chronic obstructive lung disease to live to a ripe old age. Few smokers do not use these observations to support their reluctance to give up smoking. The 'grain of truth' in this argument is that some individuals are more susceptible to the effects of tobacco smoke than others.

Increased susceptibility may originate within the individual or come from without. Genetic make-up determines outwardly obvious characteristics such as race and sex. The children of one marriage have much genetic material in common but only identical twins coming from a single fertilised egg that has divided early in its development share precisely the same genetic make-up. So in looking for genetic factors that might influence susceptibility to smoking, race, sex, family and twin studies may all have something to offer. Entwined with genetic influences there are, however, common environmental influences. Until recently most people of a given race were to be found in the same part of the world, where they would all be exposed to similar climatic and geographic influences. Members of families suffer or enjoy the same environment and share similar life styles for many years and so are jointly subject to local environmental influences. Particular value thus lies in examining migratory groups or twins who have been living apart for much of their lives. Other genetic characteristics are not externally obvious and are revealed only by close examination of the body's chemistry or an even more intimate examination of the genetic material itself within body cells. It can, however, be shown that subtle changes in body chemistry arising from genetic faults do influence susceptibility to the adverse effects of cigarette smoke.

External influences on our health are legion. Three that will be considered because they can be shown to interact adversely with smoking are diet, occupation and disease. These external influences may simply add their effect to that of smoking or the interaction may be multiplicative. With the latter the combined effects of smoking and the environmental hazard are greater than the sum of their individual effects. It should be appreciated that if very few people are exposed to a particular environmental risk, however great its effect might be, the numerical contribution to deaths will be small. On the other hand, if the number of individuals exposed is large, even a small increase in risk could have important socio-economic implications.

The incidence of smoking-related diseases clearly increases with age. This, for the most part, represents the accumulated effects of life-time exposure to cigarettes. It is, however, possible that the ability of the body to combat the damage produced by smoking could change with advancing age. Given these points, this chapter considers the evidence concerning interactions between smoking and both host and environmental factors in causing the three main smoking-related diseases: lung cancer, chronic obstructive lung disease, and coronary heart disease.

LUNG CANCER

The relation of smoking history to lung cancer is so strong that it might well be questioned whether there is any need to investigate for other risk factors. Nevertheless, some observations do hint that particular susceptibility exists.

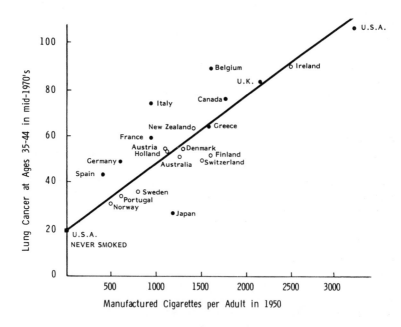

Figure 5.1. Correlation between manufactured cigarette consumption per adult in 1950 while one particular generation was entering adult life and lung cancer rates in that generation as it entered middle age in the mid-1970s [1]. Comparisons are between a wide range of developed countries
- • Rates based on over 100 deaths
- ○ Rates based on 25–100 deaths
- ▪ US non-smokers 1959–72

Race

Provided that due consideration is given to the 'generation effect' (current cancer rates are related to the smoking habits of 20–30 years earlier, not to current smoking: see Chapter 3), there is a convincing relationship between lung cancer mortality and cigarette consumption in different countries [1] (Figure 5.1). Japan is often cited as an example of a nation in which there is less lung cancer than might be predicted from cigarette consumption. Current lung cancer death rates in Japan are, however, rising steeply and this, coupled with the observation that cigarettes were virtually unobtainable in Japan during World War II, suggests that the discrepancy will not long remain substantial. Within one country, peoples of different races, but similar smoking history, do not appear to have different lung cancer mortality rates — this applies, for example, to the black and white citizens of the USA (other national statistics are reviewed in Chapter 10).

Sex

Life-time smoking habits in women differ from those in men and these (reviewed in Chapter 7) influence the development of lung cancer in women. Before World War II women smoked little and suffered little from lung cancer. Once women took up smoking habits like those of men they too, after the expected lag of a few decades, increasingly became victims of lung cancer [2,3].

In most population studies the number of non-smoking women who develop lung cancer is greater than that in non-smoking men because the number of women who are non-smokers is greater [4–6]. The position is entirely different, however, in South China and Hong Kong where the incidence of lung cancer per 100,000 non-smokers is significantly higher in women than in men [7]. One reason for this may be that women at home are unwillingly exposed to smoke produced by their husbands' smoking. The exceptionally high rates in certain populations of Chinese women, however, seem to point to some other, as yet unidentified, environmental hazard.

Genetic predisposition

There is some evidence suggesting that lung cancer may cluster in families. More lung cancer is detected in family members of patients with the disease than in the families of control subjects, but this may be at least as much due to environmental as to genetic factors.

A more subtle search for a genetic predisposition to cancer comes from enzyme studies. Some substances found in cigarette tar need to be activated within the body before they can produce cancer. One of the most extensively investigated of these is benzo-a-pyrene. It is activated by the enzyme aryl hydrocarbon hydroxylase (AHH). In the mid-1970s there was some evidence that this enzyme (AHH) was more active in patients with lung cancer, and that this function was genetically determined [8]. Subsequent experiments have rendered the situation far from clear so that a direct genetic susceptibility to the carcinogenic damage produced by cigarette smoke cannot yet be said to have been satisfactorily demonstrated [9].

Diet

Vitamin A is a substance needed by the body in small amounts to maintain the integrity of its surface membranes. Deficiency of Vitamin A is associated with dry skin, night blindness and an undue susceptibility to cancer [10]. Beta-carotene, a precursor of Vitamin A, is found in the diet in vegetables, chiefly carrots. Dietary enquiries in several populations have shown that when there is a low intake of Vitamin A and its precursors then there is about a twofold increased incidence of lung cancer [11–14]. Some of the dietary beta-carotene is converted into Vitamin A (retinol), while other retinol is absorbed directly from food. Laboratory evidence indicates that retinol will suppress cancer growth, and epidemiological studies indicate that people with above average blood retinol levels have a below average cancer risk [15]. For cancer of the lung, the evidence so far available suggests that low intake of Vitamin A increases the chance that smoking will cause this cancer. Studies to see whether increasing the dietary intake of Vitamin A can decrease the carcinogenic effects of cigarette smoking are now under way.

Lung disease as a risk factor

Localised scarring of the lungs is said to give rise to a so-called scar cancer. Widespread scarring (fibrosis) of the lungs also appears to be associated with an increased risk of lung cancer. Among patients who died from a condition known as fibrosing alveolitis, 13 per cent of 155 were found to have lung cancer [16]. Only two of these victims of lung cancer were non-smokers. Comparisons with the expected lung cancer rate in smokers in the general population indicated a 14-fold increased risk of lung cancer in cigarette smokers who also had widespread lung scarring due to fibrosing alveolitis.

Lung cancer risk and occupation

Some of the best evidence indicating a specific increased susceptibility to lung cancer comes from occupational studies [17]. Many different occupations give rise to an increased risk of lung cancer (Table 5.1), but for only two types of exposure — asbestos and radio-active decay products — has there been sufficiently adequate study of the risks in smokers and non-smokers separately to quantify the differential susceptibility.

TABLE 5.1. Occupational hazards associated with lung cancer

Minerals	:	Asbestos
		Arsenic
		Chromates
		Nickel
Chemicals	:	Chlormethyl ethers
		Coal tar distillates
		Mustard gas
Radiation	:	Uranium

Lung cancer was first directly related to asbestos exposure in 1949 [18], and since then the great excess of lung cancer in asbestos workers has been firmly established [19]. In a large group of 17,800 asbestos insulation workers there were 2,066 non-smokers. Among these were two deaths from lung cancer. By contrast in 9,590 smokers, lung cancer caused 134 deaths − a relative risk to the smoking asbestos worker of 14:1, or compared with a non-smoker outside the asbestos industry a factor perhaps of as much as 90-fold [20].

Similar observations apply to exposure to radio-active materials [21, 22]. Some of the first cases of what was later found to be lung cancer were described in workers in the Schneeberg mines (afterwards discovered to be uranium mines), long before cigarettes were invented. Data collected in Colorado on uranium mine workers suggest that the risk to non-smoking miners is small but to smokers 11 times greater − a risk 76 times that of non-smokers in the general population [23].

Reviewing trends in mortality in the United States a report by the Toxic Substances Strategy Committee of the United States (1980) concluded that large increases in lung cancer incidence were occurring over and above those attributable to smoking. Examination by Doll and Peto [1] of the data on which the conclusion was based, suggests that such an analysis is misleading and incorrect. Whilst certain occupational factors can have a dramatic effect on lung cancer incidence as indicated above, this is of importance in so few patients that it cannot influence national trends. An important observation is that lung cancer among non-smokers does not seem to have changed materially over the years, indicating that other environmental causes of lung cancer in the general population have not played an important part.

CHRONIC OBSTRUCTIVE LUNG DISEASE

As pointed out earlier (Chapter 2), apart from cancer, smoking has other harmful effects on the lungs. The excessive production of mucus, commonly called chronic bronchitis, is certainly caused by smoking and appears to afflict virtually all smokers even though they may not admit this. While it encourages recurrent respiratory tract infection, it remits when smoking is stopped and does not itself cause permanent disability.

Chronic obstructive lung disease, on the other hand, leads to disability by causing irreversible obstruction in the airways of the lungs [24]. Smoking causes airflow obstruction chiefly in two ways. The first is damage to small airways less than 2mm in diameter, and the second is emphysema, in which there is actual destruction of the walls of the air sacs in the deepest parts of the lungs [25]. Airflow obstruction appears to affect only a minority of smokers, who may therefore be unduly susceptible in some way.

Race

Geographical differences in the incidence of chronic bronchitis are closely related to environmental air pollution, and there is no evidence to suggest that racial genetic differences influence susceptibility to the propensity for smoking to produce non-malignant chronic lung disease.

Sex

The question of differing susceptibility to chronic obstructive lung disease between the two sexes has often been raised. After allowing for the effect of different smoking habits it still appears that women are to some extent protected from the adverse effects of smoking in terms of obstructive lung disease. They seem to have both fewer symptoms [26], and less emphysema [27].

Genetic predisposition

Considerable attention has been given to the potential influence of genetic factors in chronic obstructive lung disease. In 1963 Laurell and Eriksson first reported on the association between emphysema and an hereditary enzyme deficiency [28]. There are enzymes within the body which can digest protein material. These 'proteolytic' enzymes are capable of attacking the elastic tissue in the walls of the air sacs. Other enzymes oppose this destructive tendency and within the lungs the balance usually strongly favours these inhibitors. Chief amongst these is the enzyme alpha$_1$ antitrypsin (alpha$_1$ AT). A genetic fault can result in grossly deficient levels of alpha$_1$ AT. The enzyme balance in the lungs thus shifts in favour of proteolysis and lung tissue is destroyed.

Alpha$_1$ AT deficiency is associated clinically with chronic obstructive lung disease with strong emphysematous features and with onset before the age of 40 [29]. It is impossible to reverse this process, which progresses inexorably to severe respiratory disability and death. The absolute risk is difficult to determine. In one study all the men and two-thirds of the women over 40 had emphysema, but there are reports of small series of individuals with the deficiency and no lung disease [30].

Of factors which modify the development of the disease, smoking appears to be the most important. In patients with severe deficiency the age of onset of breathlessness was 35 years in smokers, and 44 years in non-smokers. Lung function at a given age was more seriously disturbed in $alpha_1$ AT-deficient smokers than in non-smokers and deteriorated faster. Atmospheric pollution did not seem to have a similar deleterious effect in $alpha_1$ AT-deficient individuals [31].

Cigarette smoking itself increases proteolytic activity in scavenger cells lodging in the lungs, so upsetting further the balance of enzymes, not only in those with $alpha_1$ AT deficiency, but also in otherwise healthy smokers. The capacity of blood scavenger cells (polymorphs) to resist the adverse effects of cigarette smoke varies widely in different individuals. This, too, is thought to be a genetically determined trait and not a secondary effect of the chronic lung disease itself [32].

The genetic abnormality for $alpha_1$ AT deficiency must be inherited from both parents before it can express itself as a low enzyme level in the blood. Considerable controversy rages concerning the possible development of emphysema in individuals who inherit the fault from just one parent. Blood levels of $alpha_1$ AT may be normal or slightly reduced [33]. The relative risk of developing chronic obstructive lung disease is probably small. The results of tests of airways function in such individuals may, however, be abnormal and some evidence is now accruing of an interaction with smoking [34,35].

There is also evidence of familial aggregation of chronic bronchitis and obstructive lung disease independent of $alpha_1$ AT deficiency [36]. Chronic respiratory disease occurs more often in children when present in both parents, and studies of identical twins with discordant smoking habits have even suggested that the genetic component was more important in determining the development of chronic obstructive lung disease than the level of smoking [37]. A precise evaluation of the quantitative risk to smokers of a genetic predisposition other than $alpha_1$ AT is, however, not yet possible.

Genetic influences might also operate in determining the lung's capacity to cope with pollutants such as cigarette smoke. Clearance of mucus from the airways has been shown by studies in twins to be genetically determined [38]. Genetic deficiency in clearance does appear to enhance the adverse effects of cigarette smoke.

ASSOCIATED DISEASES

One approach to studies to detect susceptibility to smoking is the measurement of rates of decline in airflow function over several years. This has been referred to already (see Figure 3.3). Smokers showed variable rates of decline, but a more rapid decline was likely if they already had evidence of airflow obstruction at the beginning of the study in adult life.

Various characteristics were examined for an association with a rapid decline in lung function. Neither bronchial infection nor hypersecretion of mucus appeared to be implicated, but bronchial allergy was. Though there were few overt asthmatics, the rate of decline in their lung function was steeper than for other men [24]. Furthermore, among 2,626 adults aged over 20 in Tucson, Arizona, those male smokers who reported respiratory trouble in childhood showed a faster rate of decline in lung function with age than did smokers without childhood respiratory illness [39]. So there is a hint that childhood respiratory illnesses, especially perhaps asthma, render smokers more likely to develop chronic obstructive lung disease later in life.

Environmental pollution may be specifically occupational or general, affecting an entire population. There is no definite evidence for any direct interaction in the development of obstructive lung disease between exposure to occupational dust or fumes and cigarette smoking. However, in miners, foundrymen, grain workers, cotton workers, fire fighters, and some others the effects of the two hazards appear to be additive [40,41]. In other industries the abnormalities in lung function appear to be explicable in terms of smoking habits alone. Comparisons between populations living in areas with widely different levels of non-occupational air pollution suggest that long-term exposure to high concentrations of photochemical pollutants, nitrogen dioxide, and sulphates may result in impaired lung function but that these pollutants combine with smoking in no more than an additive way [42]. There is no evidence that any form of environmental pollution or occupational exposure lessens the effects of cigarette smoking in producing chronic obstructive lung disease.

CORONARY HEART DISEASE

The situation regarding undue susceptibility to the effects of smoking is least clear in relation to coronary heart disease (CHD). Though there is rather a small increased relative risk of CHD in smokers, this is offset by the large numbers involved. The influence of smoking is, more obviously than in the other examples considered, only one of several risk factors.

The evidence suggests that the effect of smoking is at least additive to that of other factors and produces a relative risk of up to twofold or above in heavy smokers. In those with overt coronary heart disease it seems that there is seldom only one risk factor, and there is certainly interaction between risk factors. When cholesterol levels are low the effect of smoking seems relatively unimportant and the obvious risk of smoking in young middle age diminishes to insignificance in older smokers [43] (see also Chapter 4). Nonetheless the absolute increase in risk due to smoking is greater when other risk factors are high. In British civil servants the percentage of smokers dying of coronary heart disease compared with non-smokers was three times as great in those with both hypertension and raised blood cholesterol levels as in those with neither of these risk factors [44]. Perhaps the importance of such evidence lies in the ease with which these other risk factors (hypertension, raised cholesterol) can be measured so that warning of increased susceptibility to the coronary heart disease from smoking can be given to reinforce the smoker's resolve to give up smoking.

Conclusion

With a self-inflicted environmental hazard such as smoking, which has an obviously adverse effect in terms of respiratory and cardiovascular disease, it would be easy to dismiss the question of susceptibility as the vain hope of the smoker who seeks a reason for not giving up the habit. However, the evidence outlined above does suggest that some smokers may be especially at risk of developing chronic obstructive lung disease, myocardial infarction and possibly lung cancer. Even if only small numbers can be salvaged — asbestos workers from cancer, those with alpha$_1$ AT from emphysema — this is nonetheless the beginning of a contribution to the problem. And if factors can be found which reduce the increased risk — as perhaps Vitamin A therapy might in those who are deficient — the way is open for a different range of therapeutic possibilities.

References

1   Doll R, Peto R. The causes of cancer: quantitative estimates of avoidable risks of cancer in the United States today. *J Natl Cancer Inst 1981; 66:* 1193–1308

2   Doll R, Gray R, Hafner B, Peto R. Mortality in relation to smoking: 22 years' observations on female British doctors. *Br Med J 1980; 1:* 967–971

3   Jick H, Porter J, Morrison AS, Rothman KJ. Lung cancer in young women. *Arch Intern Med 1979; 139:* 745–746

4   Huhti E, Sutinen S, Reinila A et al. Lung cancer in a defined geographical area: history and histological types. *Thorax 1980; 35:* 660–667

5   Nou E, Hillderdal O. Total tobacco consumption in an unselected bronchial carcinoma population. *Eur J Respir Dis 1981; 62:* 152–159

6   Jindal SK, Malik SK, Dhand R et al. Bronchogenic carcinoma in Northern India. *Thorax 1982; 37:* 343–347

7   Chan WC, Colbourne MJ, Fung SC, Ho HC. Bronchial cancer in Hong Kong. *Br J Cancer 1979; 39:* 182–192

8   Kellerman G, Shaw CR, Luyten-Kellerman M. Aryl hydrocarbon hydroxylase inducibility and bronchogenic carcinoma. *N Engl J Med 1973; 289:* 934–937

9   Paigen B, Gurtoo HL, Minowada J et al. Questionable relation of aryl hydrocarbon hydroxylase to lung cancer risk. *N Engl J Med 1977; 297:* 346–350

10   Bollag W. Vitamin A and vitamin A acid in the prophylaxis and therapy of epithelial tumours. *International J Vitamin Research 1970; 40:* 299–314

11   Bjelke E. Dietary vitamin A and human lung cancer. *Int J Cancer 1975; 15:* 561–565

12   Hirayama T. Diet and cancer. *Nutr Cancer 1979; 1:* 67

13   Maclennan R, Da Costa J, Day NE et al. Risk factor for lung cancer in Singapore Chinese, a population with high female incidence rates. *Int J Cancer 1977; 20:* 854–860

14   Mettlin C, Graham S, Swanson MJ. Vitamin A and lung cancer. *J Natl Cancer Inst 1979; 62:* 1435–1438

15   Peto R, Doll R, Buckley JD, Sporn MB. Can dietary beta-carotene materially reduce human cancer rates? *Nature 1981; 290:* 201–208

16   Turner-Warwick M, Lebowitz M, Burrows B, Johnson A. Cryprogenic fibrosing alveolitis and lung cancer. *Thorax 1980; 35:* 496–499

17   Chovil AC. Occupational lung cancer and smoking: a review in the light of current theories of carcinogenesis. *Can Med Assoc J 1979; 121:* 548–550

18   Gloyne SR. Pneumoconiosis: a histological survey of necropsy material in 1205 cases. *Lancet 1951; i:* 810–814

19   IARC. *Working Group on the Evaluation of the Carcinogenic Risk of Chemicals to Man: Asbestos.* Lyons: International Agency for Research on Cancer. 1977: 62

20   Selikoff IJ, Hammond EC, Churg J. Asbestos exposure, smoking and neoplasia. *JAMA 1968; 204:* 106–112

21   Lundin FE, Lloyd JW, Smith EM et al. Mortality of uranium miners in relation to radiation exposure, hard-rock mining and cigarette smoking – 1950 through September 1967. *Health Phys 1969; 16:* 571–578

22   Archer VEW, Wagoner JK, Lundin FE. Uranium mining and cigarette smoking effects on man. *J Occup Med 1973; 15:* 204–211

23   Band P, Feldstein M, Saccomanno G et al. Potentiation of cigarette smoking and radiation. *Cancer 1980; 45:* 1273–1277

24   Fletcher C, Peto R, Tinker C et al. *The Natural History of Chronic Bronchitis and Emphysema.* Oxford: Oxford University Press. 1976

25   Cosio MG, Hale KA, Niewoehner DE. Morphologic and morphometric effects of prolonged cigarette smoking on the small airways. *Am Rev Respir Dis 1980; 122:* 265–271

26   Higgins MW, Keller JB, Metzner HL. Smoking, socio-economic status and chronic respiratory disease. *Am Rev Respir Dis 1977; 116:* 403–410

27   Thurlbeck WM, Ryder RC, Sternby N. A comparative study of the severity of emphysema in necropsy populations in the three different countries. *Am Rev Respir Dis 1974; 109:* 239–248

28   Laurell CB, Eriksson S. The electro-phoretic alpha$_1$ globulin pattern of serum in alpha$_1$ antitrypsin deficiency. *Scand J Clin Lab Invest 1963; 15:* 132–140

29   Kueppers F, Black LF. alpha$_1$ antitrypsin and its deficiency. *Am Rev Respir Dis 1974; 110:* 176–194

30   Eriksson S. Pulmonary emphysema and alpha$_1$ antitrypsin deficiency. *Acta Med Scand 1964; 175:* 197–205

31   Rodriguez RJ, White RR, Senior RM et al. Elastase release from human alveolar macrophages: comparison between smokers and non-smokers. *Science 1977; 198:* 313–314

32   Hopkin JM, Tomlinson VS, Jenkins RM. Variation in response to cytotoxicity of cigarette smoke. *Br Med J 1981; 283:* 1209–1212

33   Lieberman J. Heterozygous and homozygous alpha$_1$ antitrypsin deficiency in patients with pulmonary emphysema. *N Engl J Med 1969; 281:* 279–284

34   Mittman C. Editorial: The Pi mz phenotype: is it a significant risk factor for the development of chronic obstructive lung disease? *Am Rev Respir Dis 1978; 118:* 649–652

35   Madison R, Mittman C, Afifi AA et al. Risk factors for obstructive lung disease. *Am Rev Respir Dis 1981; 124:* 149–153

36   Larson RKML, Barman F, Kuepper ST et al. Genetic and environmental determinants of chronic obstructive pulmonary disease. *Ann Intern Med 1980; 72:* 627–632

37   Cederlof R. The use of twin studies in CNSLD. In Orie NGM, Van Der Lander RV, eds. *Bronchitis III.* Beaverton, Oregon: van Gorcum. International Scholarly Book Services Inc. 1971

38   Kamishima K, Yahamoto H, Shida A et al. Bronchial mucoliliary clearance in twins, smokers and non-smokers. *Am Rev Respir Dis 1982; 125:* Suppl 157

39   Burrows B, Knudson RJ, Lebowitz MD. The relationship of childhood respiratory illness to adult obstructive airway disease. *Am Rev Respir Dis 1977; 115:* 751–760

40   Sparrow D, Bosse R, Rosner R et al. The effect of occupational exposure on pulmonary function: a longitudinal evaluation of fire fighters and non-fire fighters. Five year FEV$_1$ change. *Am Rev Respir Dis 1982; 125:* 319–322

41   Detels R, Sayre JW, Coulson AM. The UCLA population studies of chronic obstructive respiratory disease. *Am Rev Respir Dis 1981; 124:* 673–680

42   Kauffman F, Drouet D, Lellouch J, Brille D. Twelve years spirometric changes amongst Paris workers. *Int J Epidemiol 1979; 6:* 201–212

43   Kannel WB, McGee D, Gordon T. A general cardiovascular risk profile. The Framingham study. *Am J Cardiol 1976; 38:* 45–56

44   Reid DD, Hamilton PJS, McCartney P et al. Smoking and other risk factors for coronary heart disease in British civil servants. *Lancet 1976; ii:* 979–981

Chapter Six

CHILDREN AND SMOKING

INTRODUCTION

Prospects for eliminating the smoking epidemic are greatest if children can be dissuaded from ever starting to smoke. This chapter will review evidence on the prevalence of smoking in children and the influences which cause them to take up and then maintain the habit. It will concentrate largely on information gathered in Britain. Much research elsewhere, particularly in Scandinavia, Australasia and the United States, supports the overall conclusions to be drawn from the British data.

Prevalence

Cigarettes enter the experience of children at an early age. Three out of four children are aware of cigarettes before they reach the age of five, whether their parents smoke or not [1]. Often children under five years have handled cigarettes and played with them in their games, and a few have actually tried to smoke a lighted cigarette, sometimes with parental encouragement. During their primary school years many more children try to smoke [2]. At 10 years of age as many as 40 per cent of boys and 28 per cent of girls have had at least a few puffs of a cigarette [3].

However, it is not until adolescence that smoking becomes a regular rather than an experimental practice. The trends evident from an earlier study of urban children from 13 Hounslow schools published in 1975 [4] have been confirmed and expanded by information from an important MRC longitudinal study of rural children in Derbyshire covering the years 1974–8 [5]. The prevalence of smoking rises steadily throughout the secondary school years. Around five to six per cent of 11-year old boys admit to smoking regularly, and by the time they reach 16, one in four are regular smokers: the figures for girls are only slightly lower [4,5]. Parallel with this rise in regular smoking are increases in the proportion of teenagers smoking occasionally (less than one cigarette a week) or experimenting with cigarettes. Figure 6.1 follows the smoking habits of a group of children of 11–12 years in 1974 till they reached school-leaving age in 1978 aged 15–16 [5]. By that time only one-quarter of these teenagers had never tried a cigarette. The recent large survey of more than 15,000 children in Cumbria and Tyne and Wear [6] confirms that in 1982, 24 per cent of 16-year olds were smoking regularly, a figure very similar to that reported for the earlier studies.

Though some earlier surveys [4,7] suggested that during the 1970s

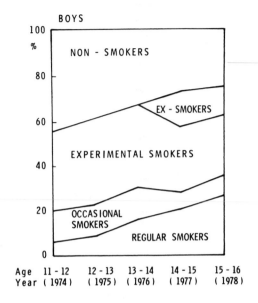

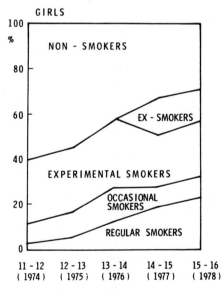

Figure 6.1. Prevalence of smoking by percentage of boys and girls separately, among Derbyshire school children followed from 1974 (when aged 11–12) till 1978 (when aged 15–16). Trends are similar in the two sexes. Whilst there is a steady increase in regular smokers (one or more cigarettes each day), the proportion of occasional and experimental smokers remains approximately constant, and the somewhat dwindling percentage of non-smokers (those who have never smoked) is added to by children who give up smoking from age 13 upwards

there was a decline in the prevalence of smoking among boys and an increase in girls, these trends were not supported by the more carefully conducted Derbyshire study [8]. This found instead that, comparing 1974 with 1977, smoking among girls became slightly less common in all age groups though there was no change in the smoking habits of boys. Among boys there was, however, a decline in the proportion who had tried smoking, so that in 1977, 54 per cent of 14−15 year olds had never had a cigarette compared with 48 per cent at the same age in 1974. These trends may, of course, not be representative of Britain as whole, and indeed a second survey of Hounslow schools in 1979 showed a falling number of regular smokers among boys, but no change in the girls [9].

The number of cigarettes smoked by teenagers who smoke regularly increases throughout adolescence. Figures from Derbyshire and Hounslow again agree closely and record around five to six per cent of 11−12 year old boys smoking more than 40 cigarettes a week, compared with 42 to 43 per cent smoking as heavily at 15 to 16 years. Figures for girls are somewhat lower, but still up to one in three girls smoke this heavily at 15 to 16 years of age.

In Hounslow 70 per cent of the regular teenaged smokers generally smoked the same brand [9]. About 85 per cent of this loyal brand group smoked middle tar cigarettes. Between 1975 and 1979 the proportion of regular smokers smoking low tar cigarettes rose from less than one per cent to six per cent. Low tar cigarettes were much more popular among experimental smokers in 1979 than in 1975, suggesting that the increased availability and acceptability of these cigarettes might encourage children to adopt smoking regularly since they would be spared the aversive physical response to stronger cigarettes in their early smoking experience.

Smoking career

Early experimentation with cigarettes tends to increase the likelihood of regular smoking when older. In Derbyshire two-thirds of those few who were regular smokers at 11 to 12 years continued to be regular smokers four years later [5]. Only nine per cent of non-smokers adopted regular smoking within the following four years. It follows that the ranks of the rather larger number of regular smokers at 15−16 years of age must have been swelled by those who in earlier years were experimental or occasional smokers. Thus the early years of adolescence are a critical period for the adoption of smoking as a regular practice.

Sociodemographic differences

Social class differences are well defined in the smoking habits of adults. Smoking is also more common among children from the households of manual workers irrespective of the parents' smoking habits [7,10]. In

Hounslow, smoking among the children of Asian and African immigrants is less common than among children who have always lived in Britain. The proportion of regular smokers among these immigrant children, especially those from Africa, increases with increasing length of time in this country [4].

Family background

Family smoking practices and attitudes have frequently been found to correlate closely with smoking by children. Young children whose mothers smoke are more likely to pretend to smoke sweet cigarettes [1]. Strong positive associations exist between adolescents' smoking practices and those of their parents [4,9,11]. Some studies [7,12] have found evidence of sex-linking in this relationship, with boys' smoking habits being similar to those of their fathers and girls' to those of their mothers.

Parental encouragement to smoke is of great importance [13]. Young smokers usually perceive their parents as being permissive about smoking [14]. In the 1982 survey from the north of England where on average 17 per cent of children were regular smokers, only eight per cent of those who thought their fathers would object had become regular smokers. By contrast 41 per cent of those who thought their fathers would not mind were regular smokers [6]. Around a quarter of 10 to 12 year old smokers reported having had their first cigarettes with their parents [2] or being given cigarettes by their parents [13]. Sadly, whilst most parents strongly disagreed with young children smoking, many expressed indifference about teenagers smoking. If a child has a brother or sister who smokes, then he or she too is more likely to become a regular smoker [6].

Family stress influences smoking habits in children. Boys whose fathers are not at home and girls whose mothers are not at home are more likely to smoke [12]. In Oxfordshire, one-parent families had a higher than expected proportion of young smokers [15], and young smokers, especially girls, were more likely to report anxiety about various problems at home [3,15].

School

Particular characteristics of the school they attend and of their teachers are factors in the recruitment of children to smoking. Girls from single-sex schools [4] and boys and girls from grammar schools [6,12] are less likely than their peers to adopt smoking. This probably reflects a more middle class background of the pupils attending grammar schools, but may also be because the teachers in those schools are less likely to smoke [15]. Boys whose teachers smoke are more likely than their peers to start smoking, especially during the first year of secondary school [16].

Adolescents who smoke tend to be disenchanted with school and eager to participate in the outside world. On average, boys who smoke perform less well academically than non-smokers [17], and children who view themselves as poor academically are more likely to smoke [18]. Teachers' views support this. Newley and Bland [19] found that non-smokers viewed smokers as foolish and lazy and that smokers were more likely than non-smokers to view themselves as foolish. Young boys and girls who smoked played truant from school more frequently [12].

Social and psychological factors

The character of children's social relationships is also an influential factor in the recruitment to smoking. The majority of young smokers' friends smoke, while the majority of non-smokers' friends do not smoke [1,4]. Over a third of young smokers report that they smoke "because their friends smoke" [2]. Peer pressure to smoke was felt by both Scottish school children [20] and by those questioned in Derbyshire [21] and in the north of England [8].

Young smokers are much more likely than their non-smoking peers to take part in mixed-sex activities such as parties and dances [6,12]. Boys and girls who smoked in Derbyshire were highly involved in social activities and also more likely to have a part-time job and to have pocket money [4,5]; whereas 51.5 per cent of one sample of adolescent smokers had a part-time job, only 17.8 per cent of their non-smoking peers had [4]. Nonetheless, 91 per cent of the children questioned in the north of England considered smoking to be a waste of money [6]. A certain eagerness to be grown-up, which Bynner [17] has called 'anticipation of adulthood', is thought to be important in recruiting adolescents to smoking, though when questioned themselves, two-thirds of young teenagers regarded it simply as 'showing off' [6].

Health effects

Though school children are now given adequate information about the health hazards of smoking, smokers appear to be less concerned and more likely to express positive attitudes towards smoking [11,13,19]. Thus 11- and 12-year olds who thought smoking a desirable habit were more likely to increase their smoking in the following year [21]. In addition, between 11 and 16 years those girls who were less aware of the health hazards were particularly at risk of becoming regular smokers [5].

Evidence has continued to accumulate of deleterious effects on the health of children who smoke. Those children who smoke report respiratory symptoms more often than their non-smoking peers irrespective of urban or rural residence [22], or of their parents' smoking practices [23]. Thirty-two per cent of regular smokers in Cumbria and the North-East had frequent coughs and 81 per cent of these children were well aware that smoking was a cause of coughing [6]. The 15 to 16-year old smokers in both Derbyshire and Hounslow who had smoked longest and who inhaled were more likely to report respiratory symptoms such as coughs, colds and shortness of breath on exertion [19,24]. It has been suggested that these figures might have been biased by young smokers being more aware of or more willing to report respiratory complaints [25]. However, independent confirmation came from the parents, who more frequently reported school absence because of cold/catarrh or bronchitis/pneumonia if their children smoked [7].

Abnormalities on clinical examination are not easy to pick up in adolescent smokers but there is objective evidence that they have impaired lung function [26] and even pathological changes in their small airways [27].

Effects of parental smoking on their children's health

Smoking by parents directly affects the health of their children. Children whose parents smoke have more respiratory symptoms and are more prone to respiratory infections than the children of non-smokers [28]. The association is particularly marked in the first year of life, when bronchitis and pneumonia are more than twice as common in infants whose parents smoke than when this is not so [29]. There is a clear link between the number of cigarettes smoked by parents and the frequency of such illnesses, which cannot be explained in terms of perinatal illness, breast feeding or poor housing or social conditions [24,30]. Maternal smoking habits are more important than paternal, and the effect is lost by three years of age, indicating that close contact is required [31]. Children who suffer such infections have clear evidence of impaired lung function by five years of age [32] and children of smoking parents are, on average, shorter than other children at primary school age by up to 1cm, after adjusting for other factors [33].

Disadvantages may persist even longer: at the age of 11, intellectual performance as revealed by reading comprehension and mathematical ability is behind that of children of non-smoking mothers by a span of six to seven months [34]. It is not clear whether this is solely a consequence of parental smoking as the child grows up, or whether it could be a delayed effect of maternal smoking during pregnancy, a topic discussed more fully in Chapter 7.

Conclusions

One of the most effective strategies in reducing the costs to health of smoking would be to stamp out the epidemic at its source – in childhood. The magnitude of the problem is self-evident and some of the causative factors in both the recruitment of children to smoking and the progress to habitual smoking have now been defined.

Within the family parental attitudes could be modified. Even the most inveterate adult smokers, though unable or unwilling to give up themselves, recognise the health hazard smoking represents for their children. Direct appeals could be made to parents to participate in actively discouraging their children from taking up smoking. It is even possible that this approach would have the useful 'side effect' of helping the parents themselves to give up the habit.

Equally importantly, teachers and educators should adopt the same role. It is indefensible for a teacher to smoke in front of a class. Health education programmes in teacher training colleges could certainly with profit be reviewed and strengthened.

Efforts to dissuade adolescents from smoking have not been conspicuously successful. Two bibliographies of health education research [35,36] reviewing the early to mid-1970s indicated that anti-smoking programmes designed for children up till that time had been largely ineffective. Few programmes have been based on a proper understanding of the factors which encourage children to smoke. It is essential that efforts are made to involve the parents (whether or not they smoke) and to change the smoking behaviour of those adults upon whom adolescents model their behaviour, as well as providing children with the knowledge and skills to resist social pressure to smoke. The success of these anti-smoking programmes will continue to be limited. Fortunately recent initiatives in this field have taken this advice and early evaluative reports give cause for guarded optimism (see Chapter 11).

On a broader front, legislation concerning the sale of cigarettes to children needs strengthening. In the 1982 survey of children from Cumbria and Tyne and Wear, 76 per cent of children under 16 years admitted that they obtained their cigarettes from shops [6]. In addition, educational campaigns designed to discourage children from smoking will continue to be limited unless they occur within a broadly supportive context. To be really effective these programmes must be accompanied by wider national action to discourage smoking, as has been the case in Scandinavia. These topics are explored more fully later in this report.

Perhaps, however, most hope for the future lies with non-smoking children. A strong enough lobby among children would influence not only their peers and juniors but also their elders, whether adolescent, teacher or parent.

References

1   Baric L. *Primary Socialisation and Smoking.* London: Health Education Council. 1979

2   Bewley BR, Bland JM. Academic performance and social factors related to cigarette smoking by schoolchildren. *Br J Preventive and Social Med 1977; 31:* 18–24

3   Murray M, Swan AV, Enock G. *A Study to Evaluate the Effectiveness of a Health Education Programme ('My Body') on Primary School Children. Report of the Second Stage of the Evaluation.* London: Submitted to Health Education Council. 1981

4   Rawbone RG, Keeling CA, Jenkins A, Guz A. Cigarette smoking among secondary schoolchildren in 1975: its prevalence and some of the factors that promote smoking. *Health Education J 1979:* 92–99
5   Murray M, Swan AV, Bewley BR, Johnson MRD. The development of smoking during adolescence – the MRC/Derbyshire smoking study. *Int J Epidemiol 1983; 12:* 3–9
6   Cancer Research Campaign News. 13 April 1983
7   Pearson R, Richardson K. The smoking habits of 16 year olds in the National Child Development Study. *Public Health 1978; 92:* 136–144
8   Bewley BR, Johnson MRD, Bland JM, Murray M. Trends in children's smoking. *Community Med 1980; 2:* 186–189
9   Rawbone RG, Guz A. Cigarette smoking among secondary schoolchildren 1975–1979. *Arch Dis Child 1982; 57:* 352–358
10   Johnson MRD, Murray M, Bewley BR et al. Social class, parents, children and smoking. *Bull Int Union Tuberc 1982; 57:* 3–11
11   Murray M, Cracknell A. Adolscents' views on smoking. *J Psychosom Res 1980; 24:* 243–251
12   Banks MH, Bewley BR, Bland JM et al. Long-term study of smoking by secondary schoolchildren. *Arch Dis Child 1978; 53:* 12–19
13   Revill J, Drury CG. An assessment of the incidence of cigarette smoking in fourth year school children and the factors leading to its establishment. *Public Health 1980; 94:* 243–260
14   Banks MH, Bewley BR, Bland JM. Adolescent attitudes to smoking: their influence on behaviour. *Int J Health Educ 1981; 24:* 39–44
15   Mangan AL. *An Investigation into Factors Underlying Cigarette Smoking Amongst 12–17 year old Children in Oxfordshire Comprehensive Schools.* London: Report submitted to Social Science Research Council. 1978
16   Bewley BR, Johnson MRD, Banks MH. Teacher's smoking. *Br J Preventive and Social Med 1979; 33:* 219–222
17   Bynner JM. *The Young Smoker.* London: HMSO. 1969
18   Bewley BR, Bland JM, Harris R. Factors associated with the starting of cigarette smoking by primary school children. *Br J Preventive and Social Med 1974; 28:* 37–44
19   Bewley BR, Bland JM. The child's image of a young smoker. *Health Education J 1978; 37:* 236–241
20   Aitken PP. Peer group pressures, parental controls and cigarette smoking among 10 to 14 year olds. *Br J Soc Clin Psychol 1980; 19:* 141–146
21   Murray M, Swan AV, Johnson MRD, Bewley BR. Some factors associated with increased risk of smoking by children. *J Child Psychol Psychiatry 1983; 24:* 223–232
22   Bewley BR, Bland JM. Smoking and respiratory symptoms in two groups of schoolchildren. *Prev Med 1976; 5:* 63–69
23   Bland JM, Bewley BR, Pollard V, Banks MH. Effects of children's and parents' smoking on respiratory symptoms. *Arch Dis Child 1978; 53:* 100–105
24   Bewley BR, Bland JM, Murray M, Swan AV. Cigarette smoking and the development of respiratory symptoms in adolescents: report of a longitudinal study. Submitted for publication
25   Bland JM, Bewley BR, Banks MH. Cigarette smoking and children's respiratory symptoms: validity of the questionnaire method. *Rev Epidemiol Sante Publique 1979; 27:* 69–76
26   Seely JE, Zuskin E, Bouhuys A. Cigarette smoking: objective evidence for lung damage in teen-agers. *Science 1971; 172:* 741–743
27   Niewoehner DE, Kleinerman J, Rice DB. Pathologic changes in the peripheral airways of young cigarette smokers. *N Engl J Med 1974; 291:* 755–758
28   Colley JRT, Holland WW, Corkhill RT. Influence of passive smoking and parental phlegm on pneumonia and bronchitis in early childhood. *Lancet 1974; ii:* 1031–1034

29   Leeder SR, Corkhill RT, Irwig LM et al. Influence of family factors on the
      incidence of lower respiratory illness during the first year. *Br J Preventive
      and Social Med 1976; 30:* 203–213
30   Leeder SR, Corkhill RT, Irwig LM et al. Influence of family factors on
      wheezing during the first years of life. *Br J Preventive and Social Med
      1976; 30:* 213–218
31   Fergusson DM, Horwood LJ, Shannon FT, Taylor B. Parental smoking and
      lower respiratory illness in the first three years of life. *J Epidemiol Com-
      munity Health 1981; 35:* 180
32   Leeder SR, Corkhill RT, Wysocki MJ et al. Influence of personal and
      family factors on ventilatory function of children. *Br J Preventive and
      Social Med 1976; 30:* 219–224
33   Rona R, Florey Cdu V, Clarke GC, Chinn S. Parental smoking at home and
      height of children. *Br Med J 1981; 2:* 1363–1365
34   Butler NR, Goldstein H. Smoking in pregnancy and subsequent child
      development. *Br Med J 1973; 4:* 573–575
35   Bell J, Billington DR. *Annotated Bibliography of Health Education Research
      Completed in Britain from 1948–1978.* Edinburgh: Scottish Health
      Education Unit. 1979
36   Gatherer A, Parfit J, Porter E, Vessey M. *Is Health Education Effective?*
      London: Health Education Council. 1979

Chapter Seven

WOMEN AND SMOKING

In recent years women have taken up smoking in increasing numbers and have begun to smoke more heavily [1]. The recognition that smoking in women is an important issue is perhaps one of the major developments in smoking research over the last decade. Although women smokers are liable to the same smoking-related diseases as are men, the magnitude of the ill-effects appeared until recently to be less definite in women. This led to the mistaken impression that women were relatively immune to the effects of smoking and many earlier investigations on smoking and health excluded women.

With the increase in cigarette consumption by women in the 1950s and 1960s (see Figure 1.1) and the greater numbers of women who acquired the habit, interest was stimulated in the harmful effects of smoking in women. In the early 1970s concern was expressed about the adverse effects of maternal smoking on the unborn child, leading to a national campaign aimed at reducing smoking among pregnant women. The hazards were described in terms of the effects of smoking on the child, rather than on the woman herself. When women began asking about particular effects of smoking on their own health, it became clear that little information was available [1]. Further interest in women and smoking was then stimulated by the discovery of the harmful effects of smoking combined with oral contraceptive use, and the United States Surgeon-General's report on smoking in 1980 was devoted entirely to the health consequences of smoking in women [2].

SMOKING TRENDS IN THE UNITED KINGDOM

Few women smoked before World War II. After that time the habit became increasingly popular, so that by 1956 some 42 per cent of women aged 16 and over were smokers [3]. Until the mid-1970s the figure remained relatively constant — fluctuating between 40 per cent and 45 per cent. There is, however, a recent indication of a definite decline in the proportion of women smoking. The General Household Survey published by the Government's Office of Population Censuses and Surveys gave a figure of 38 per cent for 1976, 37 per cent for 1978 and 1980, and just 33 per cent for 1982 [4]. The recent unpublished figures from the Tobacco Advisory Council (see Chapter 11) confirm this trend though their prevalence figure did not reach 37 per cent until 1981. This is the first time since the 1950s, when statistics were first published, that less than 40 per cent of women have been reported to be smokers.

These are encouraging findings, for the decline now seems to be affecting heavier smokers and is no longer accounted for entirely by a reduction in the number of light smokers. The percentage of women smoking more than 20 cigarettes per day was steady at 13 to 14 per cent and is now 11 per cent (1982). Even so, the average cigarette consumption per female smoker had increased from 87 cigarettes per week in 1972 to 102 in 1980 and is still, in 1982, 98 per week. This overall trend masks, however, a welcome significant decline in cigarette consumption for women aged under 25 years and over 60 as is shown in Figure 7.1. The improvement in young women is becoming as

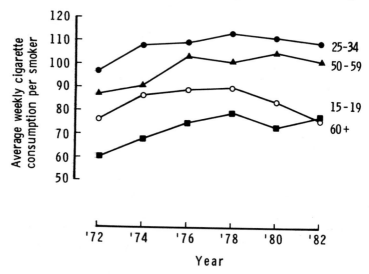

Figure 7.1. Average weekly cigarette consumption per smoker in women in five age groups. Consumption increased at all ages until 1976. Since then consumption has begun to fall in all age groups, especially the very youngest and oldest [4]

impressive as the trend in young men. The proportions of young men and women who smoke have converged and are now roughly similar (Figure 7.2). Women aged between 20 and 59 years are now the heaviest female smokers: approximately 44 per cent of them were smoking in 1980 and 39 per cent in 1982, and their average cigarette consumption continued to increase from 1972 to 1980, falling slightly in 1982.

In looking for reasons behind smoking trends in women, it is unfortunate that information relating to socio-economic status amalgamates figures for married women by their husbands' occupation with those of single women by their own occupation. Within these constraints the prevalence of smoking is highest among the wives of manual workers and lowest in the professional classes. Data on the latter may be unreliable. Anecdotally women, like men, in managerial posts are often heavy smokers [1].

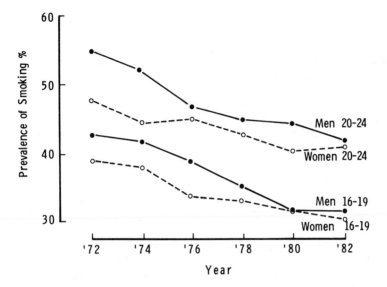

Figure 7.2. Prevalence of cigarette smoking in young men (—) and young women (- - -), illustrating the overall decline and the convergence of prevalence rates in the two sexes [4]

More reliable information comes from the health care professions. Whilst smoking is on the decline among doctors this has not been so evident among nurses. They have one of the highest smoking rates in the professional classes, at just under 50 per cent. One survey from Scotland reported in 1978 an alarming increase from 18 per cent to 60 per cent between the first and the third year of training [5]. A more recent survey from Hull gives grounds for hoping that this trend might be reversing. Between 1977 and 1982 smoking among hospital nurses fell from 48 per cent to 29 per cent [6]. Despite this, smoking among nurses still causes grave concern. The reasons why nurses smoke so heavily are not fully worked out. Though nurses are classed along with doctors as professionals in government statistics, they are more likely to come from working class homes. Yet social class alone seems insufficient to explain smoking differences. An additional factor may be stress. Nurses in psychiatric units and certain intensive care units where stress can be considerable have higher smoking rates than nurses in less stressful posts such as community care [2].

Support for the concept that smoking may be used by women (as well as men) as a means of coping with the stresses of life, comes also from the observations that women who smoke both drink more and take more mood-changing drugs than non-smoking women [2]. A formal attempt to evaluate this was made by rating a smoker's desire to smoke in situations ranging from stressful to boring [7]. Women showed a greater desire to smoke in circumstances of emotional strain or anxiety, whilst men, though more likely than women to smoke under all circumstances, showed the greatest need for cigarettes in circumstances producing boredom or fatigue.

SMOKING-RELATED DISEASES IN WOMEN

Lung cancer and other cancers

As in men, one of the strongest relationships between smoking and any particular disease is with lung cancer. The death rate from this disease increases with the number of cigarettes smoked [8]. Figure 7.3 illustrates this for British women doctors. Those who smoked more than 25 cigarettes per day had a death rate from lung cancer 30 times that of non-smoking women doctors. The relatively small risk for those smoking up to 14 cigarettes per day is due to the relatively short duration of smoking and the way the women smoked. The risk of developing lung cancer increases with the duration of smoking, the younger the age when smoking is begun and the use of plain rather than filter cigarettes [9].

An epidemic of lung cancer is now evident in women in most Western countries. In 1969 there were some 5,000 deaths from lung cancer in

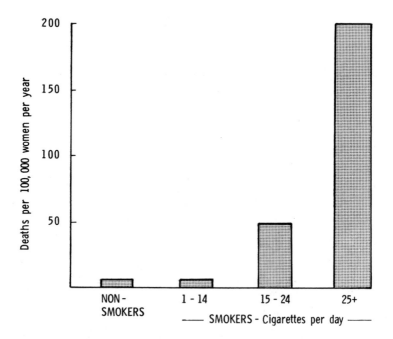

Figure 7.3. Annual age standardised death rates from lung cancer in women by daily cigarette consumption [8]. Data for 1–14 cigarettes per day are unreliable (see text)

women in England and Wales, and by 1973 the figure exceeded 6,000. Another four years later, in 1977, more than 7,000 deaths were recorded, and by 1980 there were about 8,400. This epidemic lagged several decades behind the male epidemic of lung cancer, but so did women's smoking habits. It is this generation effect, explained earlier in Chapter 3, that has given the false impression that women are not subject to smoking-related diseases to the same extent as men. But lung cancer rates in women are now catching up with those in men. In 1969 there was one female death from lung cancer to every five in men; but by 1980 the ratio of female to male lung cancer deaths had increased to one in three [9,10] (see also Figure 3.1 for detailed comparison of lung cancer deaths in men and women by age group).

Whether lung cancer rates in women will ever quite reach the proportions seen in men is debatable. Two factors are involved. First, women have until recently tended to be light smokers both in terms of the number of cigarettes smoked and to the extent which they inhale. Secondly, though women are now smoking more heavily, the cigarettes they are smoking, in this country, have relatively low tar and nicotine yields. As is discussed at greater length in Chapters 3 and 9, reducing the tar yield is associated with a reduced incidence of lung cancer as long as the number of cigarettes smoked is not increased. Given these points there is no firm evidence to suggest that women will not have an equal risk of lung cancer to men if they smoke the same type of cigarettes for the same length of time.

Cancers of the larynx, oral cavity, oesophagus, and bladder, as well as of the uterine cervix, have all been linked with smoking in women [11–14]. The reason for the association with cancer of the cervix is not clear: it may or may not be causal. In most of these conditions smoking is associated with an approximate doubling of risk.

Other lung diseases

Women smokers have an increased prevalence of productive cough, shortness of breath and wheezing when compared with non-smoking women [15]. Among British women doctors smoking was associated with an increased death rate from chronic bronchitis (Figure 7.4) and pneumonia. Although other factors, notably air pollution, play a part in the aetiology of chronic bronchitis, the condition is uncommon in non-smokers. Mortality from chronic bronchitis has been declining in England and Wales, almost certainly as a result of improvements in the control of air pollution.

ISCHAEMIC HEART DISEASE, CEREBROVASCULAR DISEASE AND OTHER CIRCULATORY DISEASES

Diseases of the circulatory system are the main cause of death in women [10] and it has been known for decades that women who

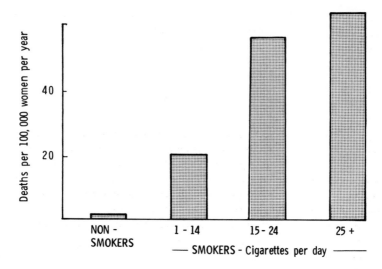

Figure 7.4. Annual age standardised death rates from chronic bronchitis and emphysema in women, by daily cigarette consumption [8]

smoke are at an increased risk of death from these conditions [16]; their mortality rate is, however, much lower than that in men. Women who smoke have, on average, about twice the incidence of death from ischaemic heart disease as have non-smokers. The incidence increases with the amount smoked and tends to be more pronounced in younger women [2].

The link between smoking and strokes in women is not so clear. Some studies have noted an increased risk [15] but others have not [14]. For one particular form of stroke which mainly occurs in young women (subarachnoid haemorrhage), however, smoking emerges consistently as a risk factor in women [17,18]. Peripheral vascular disease is also more common in women smokers than non-smokers [16].

SMOKING AND REPRODUCTION

Fertility

Smoking adversely affects reproductive function. Women who smoke are more likely to be infertile or take longer to conceive than do women who do not smoke [19,20]. In addition, smokers are more liable to have an earlier menopause than are non-smokers [21,22]. These observations point to smoking adversely affecting ovarian function, though how it does this remains unclear.

Complications of pregnancy

It is now well established that smokers who become pregnant have a small increase in the risk of spontaneous abortion, bleeding during pregnancy and the development of various placental abnormalities [23,24]. In New Zealand, Ireland and the United States there is something like a twofold increased risk of spontaneous abortion in women smoking 20 or more cigarettes a day, and this is quite independent of socio-economic, marital or other factors [2]. On the other hand, women who smoke have a lowered incidence of toxaemia of pregnancy though the advantages of this do not offset the disadvantages of smoking during pregnancy. The placenta is heavier in smoking than non-smoking women and its diameter larger [25,26]. The enlarged placenta and placental abnormalities may represent adaptations to lack of oxygen due to smoking, secondary to raised concentrations of circulating carboxyhaemoglobin (see Chapter 4).

The unborn child

It has long been recognised that the offspring of women who smoke are approximately ½lb (200gm) lighter than the offspring of women who do not smoke [27]. This observation has been confirmed in many countries. If the data are expressed as the percentage of babies weighing less than 2,500 grams (5½lb), then the figure for smokers ranges from 6.4 per cent to 17.5 per cent and for non-smokers, 3.5 per cent and 10.7 per cent, with the risk that a mother who smokes will produce a small baby being on average twice that of a non-smoker. There are clearly geographical, racial and social differences which influence the outcome of a pregnancy, but the effect of smoking is quite independent of these or any other factor concerned with the pregnancy itself [2]. The mechanism of the retardation of intrauterine growth is still debated, although it is probably due to a direct effect of some constituent of tobacco smoke, such as carbon monoxide, rather than to an indirect effect such as nutritional deficiency in smoking women [26].

The offspring of smoking women also have a small increased risk of death in the period around birth [21]. Once again, careful studies show that this risk of smoking is independent of other variables such as social class, level of education, age of mother, race or extent of antenatal care [27]. The increased risk rises to twofold or more in heavy smokers and appears to be entirely accounted for by the increased incidence of placental abnormalities and the consequences of low birthweight [28].

Suggestions that the risk of congenital abnormalities are increased have not, in general, been confirmed [29], nor have reports that the offspring of women smokers are less physically or mentally active at the time of birth [30,31]. However, there is considerable evidence that the children of mothers who smoke have certain disadvantages even up to the age of 11 years [32]. It is not clear whether these are due to the long-term effects of the mother smoking during pregnancy, or are the consequence of the mother or parents continuing to smoke as the child grows up (see Chapter 6).

Ex-smokers and women who give up smoking in the first 20 weeks of pregnancy have offspring whose birthweight is similar to that of the children of women who have never smoked. However, women receiving intensive anti-smoking advice during pregnancy did not reduce their cigarette consumption sufficiently to influence the birthweight of their offspring [33]. Why these depressing results occurred is not clear: it may be that the advice was given too late in pregnancy, or that it was ineffective in changing women's smoking despite a claimed reduction in smoking. It is hoped that different health education approaches might shed light on how to reduce the impact of maternal smoking on the unborn child.

Contraception

Women who smoke tend to favour the Pill as a method of contraception and they too bear the brunt of its ill-effects. The risk of myocardial infarction, stroke and other cardiovascular diseases in young women is

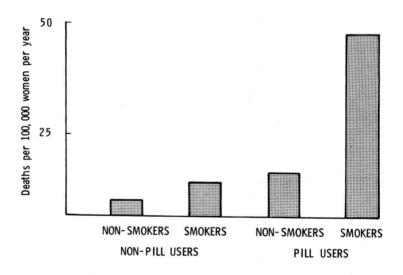

Figure 7.5. Annual age standardised death rates from coronary heart disease, stroke and other cardiovascular diseases in women according to history of smoking and oral contraceptive use [36]. The interaction between the two risk factors is illustrated

increased approximately three- to fourfold by either oral contraceptive use or by smoking [34,35]. But when the two are combined the risks multiply together leading to an approximately tenfold increase in risk overall (Figure 7.5). This effect is more marked in those over 45 years of age and somewhat less in those under 35 years [36].

Giving up

Though they are as aware of the risks of smoking as men, women find it harder to stop. They make attempts to stop as often as men and try as many different methods — but they consistently have lower success rates. This trend crosses every age group and occupation. Even when initial success rates are encouraging, women find it twice as difficult as men to remain committed non-smokers. Women left in the home whilst their husbands are out at work and children at school seem to find giving up cigarettes especially difficult. The reasons for these depressing observations are not known. Women express concern about weight gain after stopping smoking, feel they have greater stresses to combat, or need to keep their emotions in check with smoking [1], but none of these claims is properly substantiated and here is clearly an area of urgent need of research.

IMPLICATIONS FOR WOMEN

Women are as susceptible to the effects of smoking as are men and run similar risks of developing lung cancer and chronic lung disease. They are also at an increased risk of ischaemic heart disease and certain forms of stroke and peripheral vascular diseases; and their use of oral contraceptives magnifies these effects of smoking. Smoking is associated with a number of ill-effects on reproductive function — ranging from a delay in the time taken to conceive to lowering of birthweight in the offspring. Whilst ex-smokers in general have lower risks of disease than have smokers, there is little specific information available on female ex-smokers.

Although the smoking habits of young women and men are now converging, most research and anti-smoking propaganda is still aimed at and produced by men. For a variety of poorly understood reasons women find it especially difficult to give up smoking once they have begun. In the next decade still more attention needs to be given to smoking by women.

References

1   Jacobson B. *The Ladykillers: Why Smoking is a Feminist Issue.* London: Pluto Press. 1981
2   US Surgeon General. *The Health Consequences of Smoking for Women.* US Dept of Health and Human Services. 1980
3   Lee PN. *Statistics of Smoking in the United Kingdom. Tobacco Research Council Research Paper 1, 7th Edition.* London: Tobacco Research Council. 1976
4   Office of Population Censuses and Surveys. *General Household Survey: Cigarette Smoking 1972 to 1982.* Government Statistical Service GHC 83/2 July 1983
5   Small WP, Tucker L. Smoking habits of hospital nurses. *Nursing Times 1978; November:* 1878

6   Medical News. Nurses and smoking. *Br Med J 1983; 286:* 233
7   Frith CD. Smoking behaviour and its relation to the smoker's immediate experience. *Br J Soc Clin Psychol 1971; 10:* 73–78
8   Doll R, Gray R, Hafner B, Peto R. Mortality in relation to smoking: 22 years' observations in female British doctors. *Br Med J 1980; 1:* 967–971
9   Wynder EL, Covey LS, Mabuchi K. Lung cancers in women: present and future trends. *J Natl Cancer Inst 1973; 51:* 391–340
10   Office of Population Censuses and Surveys. *Mortality Statistics. Cause. 1980. Series DH2 No 7.* London: HMSO. 1982
11   Winn DM, Blot WJ, Shy CM et al. Snuff dipping and oral cancer among women in the Southern United States. *N Engl J Med 1981; 304:* 745–749
12   Wynder EL, Stellman SD. Comparative epidemiology of tobacco related cancers. *Cancer Res 1977; 37:* 4608–4622
13   Matanoski GM, Elliott EA. Bladder cancer epidemiology. *Epidemiol Rev 1981; 3:* 203–229
14   Buckley JD, Doll R, Harris RWC et al. Case-control study of the husbands of women with dysplasia or carcinoma of the cervix uteri. *Lancet 1981; ii:* 1010–1014
15   Dean G, Lee PN, Todd GF et al. Factors related to respiratory and cardiovascular symptoms in the United Kingdom. *J Epidemiol Community Health 1978; 32:* 86–96
16   Hammond EC. Smoking in relation to the death rates of one million men and women. *Natl Cancer Inst Monogr 1966; 19:* 127–204
17   Petitti DB, Wingerd J. Use of oral contraceptives, cigarette smoking and risk of subarachnoid haemorrhage. *Lancet 1978; ii:* 234–236
18   Bell BA, Symon L. Smoking and subarachnoid haemorrhage. *Br Med J 1979; 1:* 577–578
19   Tokuhata G. Smoking in relation to infertility and fetal loss. *Arch Environ Health 1968; 17:* 353–359
20   Vessey MP, Wright NH, McPherson K, Wiggins P. Fertility after stopping different methods of contraception. *Br Med J 1978; 1:* 265–267
21   Pettersson F, Fries H, Nillius SJ. Epidemiology of secondary ammenorrhea. I. Incidence and prevalence rates. *Am J Obstet Gynecol 1973; 117:* 80–86
22   Lindquist O, Bengtsson C. Menopausal age in relation to smoking. *Acta Med Scand 1979; 205:* 73–82
23   Meyer MB, Jones BS, Tonascia JA. Perinatal events associated with maternal smoking during pregnancy. *Am J Epidemiol 1976; 103:* 464–476
24   Editorial. Cigarette smoking and spontaneous abortion. *Br Med J 1978; 1:* 259–260
25   Wingerd J, Christianson R, Lovitt WV, Schoeden EJ. Placental ratio in white and black women: relation to smoking and anaemia. *Am J Obstet Gynecol 1976; 124:* 671–675
26   Naeye RL. Effects of maternal cigarette smoking on the fetus and placenta. *Br J Obstet Gynaecol 1978; 85:* 732–737
27   Butler NR, Goldstein H, Ross EM. Cigarette smoking in pregnancy and its influence on birth weight and perinatal mortality. *Br Med J 1972; 2:* 127–130
28   Editorial. Smoking and intrauterine growth. *Lancet 1979; i:* 536–537
29   Evans DR, Newcombe RG, Campbell H. Maternal smoking and congenital malformations: a population study. *Br Med J 1979; 3:* 171–173
30   Garn SM, Johnston M, Ridella SA, Petzold A. Effect of maternal cigarette smoking on Apgar score. *Am J Dis Child 1981; 135:* 503–506
31   Bosley ARJ, Newcombe RG, Dauncey ME. Maternal smoking and Apgar score. *Lancet 1981; i:* 337–338
32   Butler NR, Goldstein H. Smoking in pregnancy and subsequent child development. *Br Med J 1973; 4:* 573–575

33   Donovan JW. Randomized controlled trial of anti-smoking advice in pregnancy. *Br J Preventive and Social Med 1977; 31:* 6–12
34   Jick H, Dinan B, Rothman KJ. Oral contraceptive and non fatal myocardial infarction. *JAMA 1978; 239:* 1403–1406
35   Collaborative Group for the study of stroke in young women. Oral contraceptives and stroke in young women. *JAMA 1975; 231:* 718–722
36   Royal College of General Practitioners. Further analyses of mortality in oral contraceptive users. *Lancet 1981; i:* 541–546

Chapter Eight

BREATHING OTHER PEOPLE'S SMOKE

The three previous reports of the Royal College of Physicians on smoking and health have been concerned mainly with the effects of smoking on the smoker and the children of smokers, and how these might be reduced. Many non-smokers, however, are exposed to tobacco smoke. At home, at work, on public transport and in public places, they can scarcely avoid breathing air contaminated by other people's smoke. This mode of smoke inhalation is not actively sought: it may therefore be called involuntary or passive smoking.

To object to the unpleasant consequences of smoking is not exclusively a modern prerogative. King James I had strong words to say about the smoking habit ". . . lothesome to the eye, hateful to the nose, harmful to the braine, dangerous to the lungs, and in the black stinking fume thereof nearest resembling the horrible Stigian smoke of the pit that is bottomlesse."

Passive smoke exposure has achieved prominence recently, not only as a source of annoyance, but because of fears concerning possible health hazards. As will be evident from the contents of this chapter, it is in fact by no means easy to measure the extent of the risk to health from passive smoke exposure. Consequently, there is as yet no sure way of relating these anxieties to actual disease. Evidence is, however, being gathered about the nature of the smoke inhaled by passive smokers and the extent to which they are at risk from certain smoking-related diseases, and this will be reviewed.

Mainstream and sidestream smoke

Smoke drawn through the tobacco and taken in by the smoker is known as mainstream smoke. Smoke which arises from smouldering tobacco and passes directly into the surrounding air, whence it may be inhaled by smokers and non-smokers alike, is known as sidestream smoke. Mainstream and sidestream smoke differ in composition, partly because of the different temperatures at which they are produced. Some substances are found in greater concentrations in undiluted sidestream smoke than in undiluted mainstream smoke [1], including nicotine ($\times 2.7$), carbon monoxide ($\times 2.5$), ammonia ($\times 73$), and some carcinogens (e.g. benzo-a-pyrene $\times 3.4$). However, whereas the smoker is exposed to undiluted mainstream smoke, the sidestream smoke, to which the passive smoker is exposed, is diluted by room air to a variable extent depending on distance from the smoking source and the amount of ventilation. The room air itself contains smoke which has been inhaled and then exhaled into the air. The composition of this smoke depends on whether or not the smoker takes it into his lungs, where some constituents will be retained and others exhaled again. The concentrations of the various components of tobacco smoke breathed by the non-smoker from a smoky atmosphere are therefore extremely variable and largely unpredictable. Thus, though it is possible to express the smoke exposure of the passive smoker in terms of the number of cigarettes required to produce an equivalent amount of mainstream smoke for the smoker himself, this can be done in terms of just one constituent and then only with great uncertainty.

Carbon monoxide

Smoked in a standard way the average 1982 cigarette in the United Kingdom yields about 16–17mg of carbon monoxide in the mainstream and about 40mg in the sidestream smoke. Cigars, both regular and small, produce more carbon monoxide than cigarettes. It is a gas which mixes readily with ambient air.

The concentration of carbon monoxide produced by smoking has been measured under experimental conditions in rooms of various size [1] and in everyday social conditions [1]. Smoke-free air contains about 2.0 parts per million (ppm) of carbon monoxide. Examples of concentrations found in smoky conditions include, 7–9ppm at parties, 8–33ppm in a conference room, 40ppm in a submarine, 15–60ppm in a room, and 12–110ppm in a car. The concentrations reached depend very much on the degree of ventilation. Under ordinary social conditions with good ventilation, levels are usually below 10ppm when smokers are present and below 3ppm when they are not.

When air containing carbon monoxide is inhaled, the carbon monoxide is taken up by the blood and combines with haemoglobin to form carboxyhaemoglobin (Chapter 4). This reduces the capacity of the blood to carry oxygen. With concentrations of about 10ppm in the ambient air, the amount of carboxyhaemoglobin in the blood of a non-smoker might rise to about 2.0 per cent. After exposure to 38ppm for over an hour, the increase in carboxyhaemoglobin is about equal to that produced by smoking one cigarette [2].

Nicotine

Unlike carbon monoxide, some of the nicotine derived from cigarette smoke will settle out of the air in a room. Nicotine concentrations in the blood and urine of people exposed experimentally to smoky atmospheres [3] and in submarines [4] are increased, but are much lower than those found in smokers. About half of the non-smokers living in cities have nicotine in their blood, and most have nicotine in their urine [5]. The health consequences of this are unknown.

Carcinogens

The potent carcinogen benzo-a-pyrene is present in considerably increased amounts in the air of a smoky restaurant [6], although smoke from cooking may have accounted for some of this. In an aeroplane the levels were only slightly raised [7]. Increased levels of another carcinogen, dimethyl-nitrosamine, have been found in the ambient air of smoky public bars [8], but also in alcoholic beverages such as beer and whisky [9]. Very little is known about how much carcinogen is absorbed by a passive smoker under these circumstances, or whether these compounds, when inhaled in very low concentrations over long periods, increase the risk of developing lung cancer. However, because prolonged exposure of the cells lining the bronchi is likely to occur, it is important to look for any increase in smoking-related disease in passive smokers.

CAN PASSIVE SMOKING BE MEASURED?

It is evident from the foregoing discussion that the qualitative and quantitative contributions to the pollution of the atmosphere of enclosed spaces by smoking are extremely variable, and depend on a number of circumstances ranging from the manner of smoking to the amount of ventilation. Some substances, such as particulate matter and nicotine, slowly settle out with time, while others, such as carbon monoxide, gradually mix with the ambient air. The presence and nature of absorptive surfaces such as fabrics and hair profoundly influence the concentrations of particulate and gaseous constituents. Though both nicotine and carbon monoxide can be measured in the blood and so will give an index of exposure to these individual substances, such figures cannot be used to give a guide to exposure to other substances. Passive smoking is therefore difficult to assess quantitatively, and there are no agreed standards for expressing the extent of pollution of indoor atmospheres by tobacco smoke or its constituents.

EFFECT OF TOBACCO SMOKE ON THE GENERAL POPULATION

Most smokers do not appreciate how much their habit can annoy non-smokers [7;10–14]. The pleasure of a visit to the cinema, a meal in a restaurant, or a journey in an aeroplane, can be ruined by having to sit near to a smoker. The response of the non-smoker in such circumstances varies with the individual and his particular sensitivities, and may at times include aggressive behaviour. Discomfort can extend well beyond the period of exposure to smoke. Even one visit to a smoky environment leaves clothes reeking of smoke for days afterwards, although smokers, with their blunted sense of smell, may be less able to detect this. Similarly, a visit by a smoker to a non-smoker's home can result in a room smelling of smoke for days afterwards [15]. Fortunately, there has been some improvement in this situation as increasing numbers of restaurants, cinemas and public transport operators are recognising the right of non-smokers to breathe smoke-free air by providing non-smoking areas.

Perhaps the commonest symptoms experienced by the non-smoker in a smoky environment are irritation of the eyes [14,16] accompanied by watering, blinking and rubbing. These symptoms may be severe enough to make it impossible for the non-smoker to remain in a smoke-filled room. It is thought that acrolein is the irritant chiefly responsible for this. Irritation of the throat, cough and headache are also common in passive smokers [16]. The severity of these symptoms is related to the degree of exposure, and also to the dryness of the atmosphere. The problem may be particularly bad in places of work, where the non-smoker may not have the option of getting away from a smoky environment. The results of two surveys, one in the USA and one in Canada, suggested that about a half of non-smokers are inconvenienced by tobacco smokers at work. In some circumstances the build-up of smoke can be prevented by opening a window, but this is not always possible. Effective air-conditioning can minimise the problem by filtering out particular matter and diluting the gaseous components. However, modern recirculating systems do not remove carbon monoxide and all air-conditioning systems are expensive to run. Where possible, designation of separate smoking and non-smoking areas could be the best way of dealing with the problem.

PHYSIOLOGICAL EFFECTS

Exercise is performed less efficiently after experimental exposure to carbon monoxide levels comparable with those in a smoky environment [17,18]. The time taken to reach exhaustion is less and there is a greater increase in heart rate, effects more noticeable in older age groups. Volunteers exercising in a smoky environment showed a small decrease in lung function [19] as measured by forced expiratory flow – the ability to breathe out rapidly – and non-smokers aged 40 years and over living with smokers showed similar changes [20]. In a larger study of 2,100 middle-aged men and women [21], forced expiratory flow was highest in non-smokers working in smoke-free environments, intermediate in non-smokers who worked in smoky environments, smokers who did not inhale, and light smokers, and lowest in heavy smokers. However, the observed changes were small and the study has been strongly criticised [22,23] on both technical and methodological grounds, and in the selection of the sub-groups. Furthermore, other studies have not supported these findings [24,25] and it is not yet known whether such small changes in function are associated with increased morbidity or mortality in passive smokers.

Various driving skills are adversely affected by levels of carboxy-haemoglobin equal to those found in passive smokers [26]. Vision during driving is also affected, including colour vision, peripheral vision, brightness discrimination and recovery from glare [27]. The effects on driving are, however, relatively small, and their potential significance in relation to road safety unexplored.

LUNG CANCER

Although much work has been done on the production of cancer in experimental animals using high doses of carcinogens, very little is known about the effects on man of exposure to low doses over a long period of time. In particular, it is not known whether there is a threshold dosage, below which carcinogenesis does not occur, or whether exposure to any dosage will increase the risk of developing cancer. If the latter theory is correct, then this is a good reason for suspecting that passive smoking may increase the risk of lung cancer.

Four studies describing investigations of the incidence of lung cancer in passive smokers have been published. Two, one from Japan and one from Greece, reported an increase in lung cancer in the non-smoking wives of men who were smokers, while the other two, one from Hong Kong and one from the USA, failed to demonstrate any such relationship. It should be pointed out that neither the American or the Japanese studies were designed to answer this particular question.

The Japanese study

In this study, 91,540 non-smoking wives and 17,366 who smoked, aged 40 and over, were interviewed and then followed up for 14 years [28]. The incidence of lung cancer in non-smoking wives whose husbands smoked 20 or more cigarettes a day, compared with the risk in those whose husbands did not smoke (the risk ratio) was 2.08. In those whose husbands smoked fewer than 20 cigarettes a day, or were ex-smokers, the risk ratio was 1.6. These results should be compared with the risk ratio of lung cancer in all Japanese women who smoke of about 3.8 and in heavy smokers of about 5. Urban living could not account for the findings because the effects of passive smoking were even more marked in the wives of agricultural workers. Other forms of cancer and ischaemic heart disease were not affected by the husbands' smoking habits. This study has aroused much comment, but the criticisms that have been made were on matters of technical detail and do not invalidate the main conclusions. Interested readers should refer to the original paper and the correspondence which followed [29]. Despite undoubted problems with the statistical methodology, a puzzling excess of lung cancer in the non-smoking wives of smoking men compared with those of non-smoking men persists. These findings indicate the need for further research.

The Greek study

Fifty-one women admitted to hospital suffering from lung cancer, and 163 women admitted for other reasons, were compared with respect both to their own and their husbands' smoking habits [30]. The risk ratio for lung cancer in non-smoking women whose husbands smoked up to 20 cigarettes a day was 2.4, and in those whose husbands smoked more than 20 cigarettes a day, 3.4. The control group appeared to be a good match, except that it contained a greater proportion of women who had never married. When they were excluded from the statistical analysis, the finding of an increased risk in passive smokers remained. Although the Greek study was based on only a few cases, the results are in line with those of the Japanese study. Further work with larger groups is required to substantiate the findings.

The American study

The data on which this is based were gathered as part of a prospective, continuing study by the American Cancer Society. It is much larger than the other studies, and as such its results carry more weight. There were 176,739 non-smoking women included in the study, who were followed for a period of 12 years [31]. The risk ratio for non-smoking wives whose husbands smoked fewer than 20 cigarettes a day was 1.37, but for those whose husbands smoked 20 or more a day it was only 1.04. Neither of these ratios is statistically significant. Nevertheless, the differences are in the same direction as in the Greek and Japanese studies [28,30], and overall the three sets of results are consistent with a 50 per cent increase in lung cancer in the non-smoking wives of husbands who smoke [32] (Figure 8.1). It is important to grasp the overall significance of this for British women. Because lung cancer in this country is uncommon in women who do not smoke, it would represent only a small absolute excess of approximately two cases per 100,000 non-smokers per year.

It is interesting to speculate as to the reasons why the American and Japanese studies differed in their findings. These might include (1) different methodology; (2) a higher proportion of female office workers in the USA; (3) a higher divorce rate in the USA, making the smoking history of the ex-husband relevant; (4) smaller size of rooms in Japan; (5) different social customs; (6) husbands who smoke mainly at work; and (7) non-smoking wives who meet smokers in or outside the house.

The Hong Kong study

Two hundred and thirty-three patients, all married women who were non-smokers were studied. Of the 84 who had lung cancer, 40.5 per cent lived with husbands who were smokers, while of the 139 'comparable' control patients, 47.5 per cent lived with husbands who smoked.

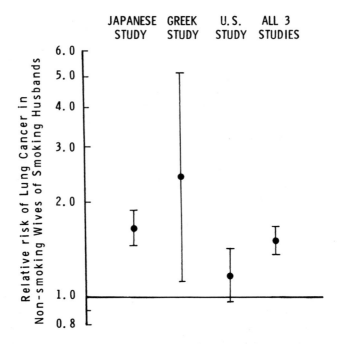

Figure 8.1. The relative risk of developing lung cancer in the non-smoking wives of husbands who smoke compared with other non-smoking women. The figure is based on revised estimates of risk as calculated in reference 29, so that figures differ slightly from those given in the text. An estimate of the overall risk from the three studies is given

Thus no excess of lung cancer in the women passively exposed to smoke was demonstrated [33]. Details of the study are lacking in this brief report, so that its validity is difficult to judge, and there is reason to believe that some other environmental factor is responsible for the high lung cancer rate in non-smoking women in Hong Kong (see also Chapter 5).

Children

The effects of passive smoking on the unborn child and on the children of parents who smoke are described elsewhere in this report (Chapters 6 and 7) and are important issues to be considered in an overall analysis of the dangers of breathing other people's smoke.

Effects of passive smoking on those suffering from disease

When healthy people breathe air containing carbon monoxide, the loss of oxygen-carrying capacity resulting from the formation of carboxy-haemoglobin is probably insufficient to affect the functioning of the heart. In the presence of heart disease, however, it may well be sufficient to make symptoms worse. When exposed to low levels of carbon monoxide [34,35] or cigarette smoke [36], patients with coronary heart disease cannot exercise for as long before being stopped by angina, and they increase their pulse rate and blood pressure more quickly. Patients with chronic obstructive lung disease similarly find their exercise tolerance reduced by exposure to carbon monoxide [37].

True allergy to tobacco is rare. However, patients with asthma or other allergic diseases seem to be more likely to find tobacco smoke irritating. Lung function studies in asthmatic subjects exposed to tobacco smoke have given conflicting results. Though one group showed reduced forced expiratory flows [38], another failed to demonstrate any such change, even though wheeziness and tightness in the chest were present [39].

Vascular disease is well recognised in smokers, and there is an interesting report of the occurrence of Raynaud's disease (spasm of the small arteries of the fingers) in the two successive wives of a heavy smoker. The first was relieved of her symptoms by separation from her husband, and the second by separation from the smoky environment [40].

Further research

Though the health consequences of smoking have been under investigation since the 1930s, the effects of passive smoking by adults have become the subject of research only relatively recently. Thus the weight of accumulated evidence regarding its possible harmful effects is much less than is the case with active smoking. Further uncertainty arises because the degree of exposure to smoke is less in passive smoking than in active smoking, so that the harmful effects may be more difficult to detect. To show statistically significant effects, larger and carefully conducted prospective studies will be required. The great difficulties inherent in the measurement of passive smoking have already been alluded to. To obtain meaningful conclusions from future studies, effective methods of measurement need to be developed.

Conclusion

The adverse social consequences of passive smoke exposure have come increasingly into prominence, first, as other sources of air pollution have come under control, and, secondly, as the serious health effects of smoking on the smoker have been increasingly widely perceived.

Although the extent to which passive smoke exposure can damage the health of otherwise healthy individuals is by no means clear, there is already sufficient evidence as to the discomfort and annoyance that breathing other people's smoke can cause. Non-smokers at work and play, in transport and in public places should have the right to choose not to be so exposed.

References

1   US Department of Health, Education and Welfare. *Smoking and Health.* DHEW Publication No (PHS) 79-50066. 1979
2   Russell MAH, Cole PV, Brown E. Absorption by non-smokers of carbon monoxide from room air polluted by tobacco smoke. *Lancet 1973; i:* 576–579
3   Harke H-P. The problem of "passive smoking". *Dtsch Med Wochenschr 1970; 112:* 2328–2334
4   Cano JP. Catalin J, Badre R et al. Determination de la nicotine par chromatographie enphase gazeuse. II. Applications. *Ann Pharm Fr 1970; 28:* 633–640
5   Russell MAH, Feyerabend C. Blood and urinary nicotine in non-smokers. *Lancet 1975; i:* 179–181
6   Galuskinova V. 3,4-Benzpyrene determination in the smoky atmosphere of social meeting rooms and restaurants. A contribution to the problem of the noxiousness of so-called passive smoking. *Neoplasma 1964; 11:* 456–458
7   National Institute for Occupational Safety and Health. Department of Transportation, Federal Aviation Administration. *Health Aspects of Smoking in Transport Aircraft.* US Department of Health, Education and Welfare, Public Health Service, Health Services and Mental Health Administration, National Institute for Occupational Safety and Health, Divisions of Technical Services. 1971
8   Brunnemann KD, Hoffman D. Chemical studies on tobacco smoke. LIX. Analysis of volatile nitrosamines in tobacco smoke and polluted indoor environments. In Walker FA, Castergnaro M, Griciute L, Lyle RE, eds. *Environmental Aspects of N-Nitroso Compounds.* Lyons: International Agency for Research on Cancer Publication No. 19. 1978: 343–356
9   Walker EA, Castagnaro M, Garren L et al. Intake of volatile nitrosamines from consumption of alcohols. *J Natl Cancer Inst 1979; 63:* 947–951
10   National Clearing House for Smoking and Health. *Adult Use of Tobacco.* US Department of Health, Education and Welfare, Public Health Service. DHEW publication HSM 73-8727. 1973
11   Shephard RJ, Labarre R. *Attitudes to Smoking and Cigarette Smoke. The Toronto Survey.* Toronto: University of Toronto. 1976
12   Speer F. Tobacco and the non-smoker. A study of subjective symptoms. *Arch Environ Health 1981; 36:* 443–446
13   Weber A, Fischer T. Passive smoking at work. *Int Arch Environ Health 1980; 47:* 209–221
14   Weber A, Fischer T, Grandjean E. Passive smoking in experimental and field conditions. *Environ Res 1979; 20:* 205–216
15   Artho A, Kock R. Caracterisation olfactive des composes de la fumee de cigarettes. *Ann du Tabac 1973; section 1–11:* 37–45
16   Weber A, Jermini C, Grandjean E. Irritating effects on man of air pollution due to cigarette smoke. *Am J Public Health 1976; 66:* 672–676
17   Aronow WS, Cassidy J. Effect of carbon monoxide on maximal treadmill exercise. A study in normal persons. *Ann Intern Med 1975; 83:* 496–499
18   Gliner JA, Raven PB, Horvath SM et al. Man's physiologic response to long-term work during thermal and pollutant stress. *J Appl Physiol 1975; 39:* 628–632
19   Shephard RJ, Collins R, Silverman F. Response of exercising subjects to acute 'passive' cigarette smoke exposure. *Environ Res 1979; 19:* 279–291
20   Kauffmann F, Perdrizet S. Effect of passive smoking on respiratory function. *Eur J Respir Dis 1981; 62:* Suppl 11: 109–110
21   White JR, Froeb H. Small-airways dysfunction in non-smokers chronically exposed to tobacco smoke. *N Engl J Med 1980; 302:* 720–723

22   Lee PN. Passive smoking. *Food and Chemical Toxicology 1982; 20:* 223–229
23   Adlkofer F, Scherer G, Weimann H. Small airways dysfunction in passive smokers. *N Engl J Med 1980; 303:* 392–394
24   Pimm PE, Silvermann F, Shephard RJ. Physiological effects of acute passive exposure to cigarette smoke. *Arch Environ Health 1978; 33:* 201–213
25   Schilling RSF, Letai AD, Hui SL et al. Lung function, respiratory disease, and smoking in families. *Am J Epidemiol 1977; 106:* 274–283
26   Ray AM, Rockwell TH. An exploratory study of automobile driving performance under the influence of low levels of carboxyhaemoglobin. *Ann NY Acad Sci 1970; 174:* 396–408
27   Yabroff I, Meyers E, Fend V et al. *The Role of Atmospheric Carbon Monoxide in Vehicle Accidents.* Menlo Park, California: Stanford Research Institute. 1974
28   Hirayama T. Non-smoking wives of heavy smokers have a higher risk of lung cancer: a study from Japan. *Br Med J 1981; 282:* 183–185
29   Correspondence. Non-smoking wives of heavy smokers have a higher risk of lung cancer. *Br Med J 1981; 282:* 985, 1156, 1393–1394; *283:* 914–917, 1464–1466
30   Trichopoulos D, Kalandidi A, Sparros L, MacMahon B. Lung cancer and passive smoking. *Int J Cancer 1981; 27:* 1–4
31   Garfinkel L. Time trends in lung cancer mortality among non-smokers, with a note on passive smoking. *J Natl Cancer Inst 1981; 66:* 1061–1066
32   Hirayama T. Letter. *Br Med J 1981; 283:* 916–917
33   Chan WC. Figures from Hong Kong. *Dtsch Med Wochenschr 1982; 124:* 16
34   Anderson EW, Andelman RJ, Strauch JM et al. Effect of low-level carbon monoxide exposure on onset and duration of angina pectoris. A study of ten patients with ischemic heart disease. *Ann Intern Med 1973; 79:* 46–50
35   Aronow WS, Ishell MW. Carbon monoxide effect on exercise-induced angina pectoris. *Ann Intern Med 1973; 79:* 392–395
36   Aronow WS. Effects of passive smoking on angina pectoris. *N Engl J Med 1978; 299:* 21–24
37   Aronow WS, Ferlinz J, Glauser F. Effect of carbon monoxide on exercise performance in chronic obstructive pulmonary disease. *Am J Med 1977; 63:* 904–908
38   Dahms TE, Bolin JF, Slavin RG. Passive smoking. Effects on bronchial asthma. *Chest 1981; 80:* 530–534
39   Shephard RJ, Collins R, Silverman F. "Passive" exposure of asthmatic subjects to cigarette smoke. *Environ Res 1979; 20:* 392–402
40   Bocanegra TS, Espinosa LR. Raynaud's phenomenon in passive smokers. Letter. *N Engl J Med 1980; 303:* 1464–1466

Chapter 9

LESS DANGEROUS FORMS OF SMOKING?

Despite all that has been done by education and propaganda, people continue to smoke cigarettes. In setting out to examine the claims for less dangerous forms of smoking, we wish to underline from the outset that the top priority is to persuade smokers to give up smoking. Smoking cessation is indeed possible for very large numbers of people. There are at least eight million ex-smokers in the United Kingdom and 33 million in the USA. Yet some smokers cannot give up and others will not. Thus, though falling short of the ideal of a smoking-free society, it is worthwhile considering ways in which the smoker can have the tobacco he craves in a less dangerous form.

Smoking pipes or cigars might be one way of achieving this end. The total death rates among men who have smoked only pipes are not significantly greater than those of non-smokers, and cigar smokers have only a modest increase in risk of premature death [1]. The most likely explanation of this relative immunity is that nicotine is absorbed from the alkaline smoke in the mouth so that smokers of pipes need not inhale. But a switch from cigarettes to pipes would benefit only some smokers, for once smokers have experienced the special pattern of nicotine absorption that comes from inhaling cigarette smoke, they usually continue to inhale after switching to pipes or cigars, and consequently would probably derive little benefit from the change [2]. It would not be easy, nor would it indeed be desirable in any way to persuade children who take up smoking to adopt a form of smoking different from that of adults.

One possibility that does not seem to have been explored is the development of a cigarette with less acid or even alkaline smoke which, like pipe smoke, would allow nicotine to be absorbed in the mouth and discourage inhalation.

To substitute taking dry snuff for smoking cigarettes would be another possible solution for a few individuals, since snuff takers absorb nicotine from their noses in a pattern not very different from that of cigarette smokers from their lungs [3]. Unfortunately, although there are said to be 500,000 snuff takers in Britain, no survey has yet been made of any diseases to which they may be liable. Since there are carcinogens in snuff there might be an excess of nasal cancer. It is certainly recognised that those who chew tobacco or hold wet snuff in their mouths (snuff dipping) have an increased risk of cancer of the mouth [3]. From a practical viewpoint, however, even if the adverse effects were only slight, it is hard to believe that a massive switch from cigarette smoking to snuff taking could be brought about, or that it would be acceptable to smokers.

REDUCING THE HARMFUL COMPONENTS
OF CIGARETTE SMOKE

Since the incidence of all the main diseases caused by smoking shows a quantitative relationship with life-time exposure to cigarette smoke, reduction of the smokers' exposure to the constituents of the smoke which are thought to cause these diseases should lower their incidence.

Since the role of cigarette tars in the causation of cancer of the lung has for long been much clearer than the role of any component of cigarette smoke in causing cardiovascular or respiratory diseases, attention has been concentrated on developing lower tar cigarettes. This has been done by using different varieties of tobacco, by curing it in different ways, by the use of filters, and by increasing the porosity of the paper so that the smoke is diluted by air taken in as the smoker draws on his cigarette. Loss of flavour of the smoke can be compensated for by adding flavouring to the cigarettes [4,5] (though there is no means of predicting whether or not this too might be hazardous to health).

Changes in the sales-weighted yields of British cigarettes are shown in Figure 9.1 [6,7]. Tar yields remained high until the late 1950s, but thereafter there has been a steep and continuing decline in the sales-weighted tar yields, from 30.4mg per cigarette in the period 1955–1961 to 15.0mg in 1982, a drop of half.

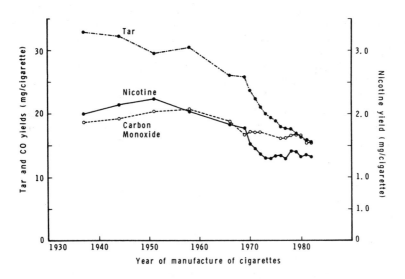

Figure 9.1. Average sales-weighted yields of tar, nicotine and carbon monoxide for British cigarettes from approximately 1960 onwards. Detailed annual figures are available only after 1969

Coincidentally with the reduction in tar, there have been reductions in nicotine and to a lesser extent carbon monoxide yields. The fall in nicotine was from 2.03mg in 1955–1961 to 1.28mg in 1974 (37%) but since then the level has risen slightly (to 1.39mg) in 1979. The trend for carbon monoxide has been rather less than that for nicotine, falling from 20.6mg to 16.0mg per cigarette (22%) in 1976 with a subsequent small rise (to 16.6mg) in 1979. These recent rises are due to increased sales of king-size cigarettes.

EFFECTS OF INTRODUCTION OF LOWER TAR/NICOTINE CIGARETTES ON INCIDENCE OF SMOKING-RELATED DISEASES

Chapter 2 reviewed evidence relating to changes in smoking habits which take place when smokers switch to lower tar/nicotine yield cigarettes. It was shown that when smokers change to lower yield cigarettes they do not compensate completely for the loss of nicotine by smoking an appropriate additional number of cigarettes. Thus they have a lower exposure to all smoke constituents. This being so we should now be able to observe some reduction in the incidence of smoking-related diseases consequent upon the lower deliveries of tar, nicotine, and perhaps carbon monoxide in recent years.

There are two main sources of evidence by which the effects of smoking lower tar cigarettes on health can be measured.

The first is from specific surveys of the incidence of or death rates from smoking-related diseases in smokers of different types of cigarettes. The major difficulty of interpreting such surveys is that it is not possible to compare long-term users of high tar cigarettes with long-term users of low tar cigarettes, partly because the changes are recent and partly because smokers vary the type of cigarettes which they smoke. Furthermore, people who have decided to smoke lower tar/nicotine cigarettes are not a random sample of all smokers. They may have made the change because they are more concerned with their health and may have adopted other beneficial habits such as changes in diet, amount of exercise, or being more scrupulous in treating conditions such as high blood pressure or diabetes. They may also have made the change from higher tar/nicotine cigarettes because they are less addicted to nicotine than smokers who have not changed and may therefore inhale less, leave longer stubs, take fewer puffs from each cigarette, and so on. For these reasons they may be people who would in any case have been less liable to smoking-related diseases and have better health prospects than those who keep to high tar/nicotine cigarettes.

Secondly, there are national death rates, and in particular the national death rates in early middle age, where smokers have had the greatest change in life-long average tar deliveries. Trends in national death rates are free from self-selection bias, of course, for they reflect changes in death rates of all smokers, who comprise 40–50 per cent of the population. Thus so long as there has been no large change in the number of cigarettes smoked per adult (and this was true of men in the United Kingdom for the years 1950–1975) these figures will reflect effects due to changes in cigarette composition. If the fall of tar/nicotine delivery of cigarettes is responsible for reducing deaths from smoking-related diseases, national death rates from these diseases should fall after an appropriate interval. These overall death rates, however, may be influenced by other changes coincident with the fall in tar/nicotine delivery such as improvements in diagnosis, treatment or general environmental changes. With these reservations in mind we can look at the evidence in respect of total death rates (which are at least free from any diagnostic bias) and of death rates from the three major disorders – lung cancer, coronary disease and chronic obstructive lung disease.

Total death rates in population samples

The most important source of such evidence comes from a study of one million American men and women whose smoking habits were first recorded in 1959–60 and subsequently recorded every two years [8]. Brands of cigarettes smoked were recorded so that the tar yields were known. These were related to deaths during the first six years of the study. Rates for those smoking high and low yielding cigarettes are shown in Figure 9.2 and are compared with death rates of non-smokers. Smokers of low tar/nicotine cigarettes, both men and women, had roughly 15 per cent lower death rates than smokers of tar/nicotine

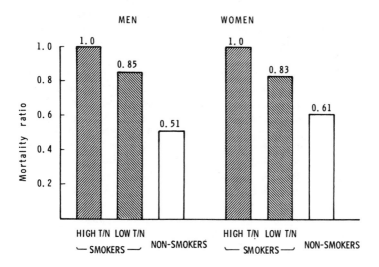

Figure 9.2. Mortality ratios in men and women for deaths from all causes, for non-smokers and smokers of high and low tar/nicotine yield, the figures being adjusted to give a mortality ratio of 1.0 for those smoking high tar/nicotine cigarettes

cigarettes; non-smokers had death rates about 50 per cent lower. This certainly suggests that smoking cigarettes with lower yields may be less dangerous than smoking high tar/nicotine cigarettes, but for the reasons given above the differences could at least in part be attributable to differences in self care between those who did and those who did not change to lower tar/nicotine cigarettes.

Lung cancer

Specific surveys

Comparisons between types of cigarettes smoked by hospital patients with lung cancer and by control patients [9—11] have indicated that smokers of filter cigarettes (which tend to give low tar delivery) have a lower risk of lung cancer than smokers of plain cigarettes. In the major American prospective study, referred to above, the lung cancer rate in male smokers of low tar cigarettes was 80 per cent and the female rate was 60 per cent of that in the corresponding high tar smokers. In non-smokers the male rate was seven per cent and the female rate 22 per cent of the high tar rate*. The results of this study, therefore, imply that there is a moderate reduction of lung cancer risk in both sexes associated with smoking lower tar/nicotine cigarettes, while in non-smokers the risk is extremely small.

A study of microscopic changes in the bronchial tubes of 211 men in New Jersey who had died of causes other than lung cancer in 1955—60 reported the presence of precancerous changes ('carcinoma in situ') in cigarette smokers which were absent in non-smokers. The percentage of samples showing these severe changes ranged from 2.6 per cent in light smokers to 22.5 per cent in heavy smokers. The study was repeated on 234 men who died in 1970—77 to see how much the fall in tar delivery of cigarettes smoked between the studies had affected the abnormalities in the lungs [12]. The frequency of severe changes had fallen to 0.1 per cent in light smokers and 2.2 per cent in heavy smokers. It is surprising that such a large change could have occurred as a result of the 30 per cent lowering of mean tar delivery of US cigarettes between the two periods. It is also difficult to interpret the meaning of these observations, for there has been no corresponding decline in deaths from lung cancer in the United States since the first period, so that the precancerous changes cannot have been immediate predictors of the development of lung cancer. But the study does indicate that the changes in types of cigarette smoked after 1960 did result in less damage to the lining of the bronchial tubes.

---

* This contrast between the two sexes may be due to the women's lung cancer rate being much lower than the male rate, so that an uncommon type of lung cancer, unrelated to smoking, is more frequent among women. See also Chapter 5.

Changes in national lung cancer deaths

As pointed out earlier (Figure 3.1) there has been an important down-ward trend in lung cancer mortality in men of all ages in the United Kingdom. In women this trend has been seen only in the youngest age groups. In seeking an explanation for these trends the influence of smoking habits 20–30 years earlier has been shown to be of paramount importance (the 'generation effect').

There is no obvious explanation for these falls in national lung cancer death rates other than the changes in the tar delivery of cigarettes. Cigarette consumption per head did not begin to fall in men until very recently (see Figure 11.2). If the fall in lung cancer deaths is due to smoking lower tar/nicotine cigarettes, complete compensation for the lower nicotine by increasing total smoke intake cannot have been wide-spread. Declining air pollution is unlikely to have contributed much to this effect since air pollution appears to have little if any effect on lung cancer incidence [13], and moreover similar decreases have been observed in unpolluted Finland [13].

In the USA, although there have been similar changes in the tar delivery of cigarettes, there has been only a small and recent reduction in lung cancer death rates, confined to men under 50. This is probably because any possible effect due to reduced tar delivery is swamped by the 'generation effect' in the USA, for the onset of widespread cigarette smoking by young men probably occurred later there than in the United Kingdom [13]. This may also be responsible for the relatively small effect of low tar/nicotine smoking on lung cancer deaths in the large American prospective study, which was confined to men and women over the age of 40 [11]. But a more important consideration is simply that these studies were done in the 1960s, when tar reductions were less extreme than they now are and when even middle-aged smokers of low tar cigarettes had actually smoked high tar cigarettes for most of their smoking lives.

The British national death rates from lung cancer thus probably pro-vide a better index of what may be expected from further reductions in the tar delivery of cigarettes in respect of lung cancer deaths than do the American figures, which are so distorted by the 'generation' effect. In the future, however, the influence of falling cigarette consumption will also need to be taken into consideration.

Chronic bronchitis and chronic obstructive lung disease

Three studies have now looked at the relationship between the type of cigarettes smoked and the development of bronchitis and airways obstruction. In two of these [14,15] smokers of low tar cigarettes were shown to have significantly less productive cough than smokers of higher tar cigarettes, but these benefits were much smaller than the benefits from reduction in the amount smoked, and stopping smoking had a still larger effect. A British necropsy study suggested a halving of bronchitis deaths in smokers of filter cigarettes, but this study has been criticised as liable to bias [16]. The question of rate of loss of lung function and cigarette tar content is less clear. Two studies [14,17] suggest that low tar cigarettes do not lessen the rate of decline, though the interpretation of the data in the first of these has been criticised [18].

Changes in death certification rates from chronic obstructive lung disease are very difficult to interpret. In the United Kingdom during the period 1930–50, when death certification rates from lung cancer were increasing rapidly (especially in men), those from 'bronchitis' remained constant in men and fell in women. Since then the male 'bronchitis' rates have fallen remarkably steeply and the female rates less so. These changes may be attributable to declining air pollution following the 1956 Clean Air Act, but this is not known for certain. Although air pollution has little absolute effect on chronic obstructive lung disease mortality in non-smokers, it might, at least in theory, modify the harmfulness of tobacco. A second factor that might modify the effects of tobacco on chronic obstructive lung disease is the general improvement in living standards over the past half-century. Even before the first (1962) Royal College of Physicians report on smoking, when there was much less difference in cigarette usage between social classes, people in social class I were six or seven times less susceptible to chronic obstructive lung disease than those in social class V (see also Chapter 3).

Despite these difficulties (and those produced by changing conventions in death certification), the national trends in chronic obstructive lung disease mortality in middle age are of some interest, and they are presented for men in Table 9.1. Similar trends are seen in women,

TABLE 9.1. Death certification rates per million from chronic obstructive lung disease in men in England and Wales

Age	1966–70	1976–80	Ratio $\dfrac{1976-80}{1966-70}$
35–44	44	19	0.4
45–54	330	170	0.5
55–64	1,745	953	0.5
65–74	5,653	3,600	0.6
75–84	10,396	9,684	0.9

This table utilises the 9th International classification of Disease categories 491–2, 496 and 518–9 which includes chronic bronchitis, chronic obstructive lung disease and a small number of allied conditions. Figures for those over 65 are potentially unreliable because of errors in death certification.

though overall rates are much lower. The pattern is encouragingly similar to that seen for lung cancer [13] with substantial decreases beginning to emerge among men throughout middle age and among women in early middle age. The lack of decrease among women in later middle age might be, as for lung cancer, because of the effects of delayed adoption of smoking by women in earlier decades. These encouraging downward trends are consistent with the suggestion that the large decreases in tar deliveries of cigarettes over the past quarter century have substantially reduced the rate of development of chronic obstructive lung disease. Thus, although they fall far short of proof of this suggestion, they should at least prevent the converse suggestion that it is unwise to press for tar level reductions "because they will have no effect, or even an adverse effect, on chronic obstructive lung disease".

Coronary heart disease

Several studies have compared coronary heart disease in smokers of filter cigarettes and plain cigarettes [19,20] and, apart from one study in the United Kingdom (which has been heavily criticised in respect of its design), the effect has been negligible. In the Framingham prospective study [19], coronary deaths were about 10 per cent lower in male smokers of low tar/nicotine cigarettes compared with those in smokers of high tar cigarettes; the reduction in women was 20 per cent. In non-smokers the death rates in both sexes were about half of those in smokers of high tar cigarettes. A further study recently published was again negative [21]. Non-fatal first myocardial infarctions were no fewer in young men aged 30–54 years who smoked cigarettes with reduced amounts of nicotine and carbon monoxide than in those who smoked other brands.

It is exceedingly difficult to deduce precise information on the effects of changing the tar, nicotine or carbon monoxide yields of cigarettes on coronary heart disease from available figures, for smoking is only one among many factors which may affect death rates from this disease. In the United States there has been a consistent overall fall in deaths from coronary heart disease over the past 20 years, a trend only just becoming evident in the United Kingdom [22]. There have also been considerable improvements in the detection and treatment of high blood pressure, and changes have occurred in food consumption (especially a lowering of the intake of saturated fats) and many people have been taking more vigorous exercise.

The effects of lower tar/nicotine cigarettes on pregnant mothers

The harmful effects of smoking during pregnancy have been catalogued in Chapter 7. There is no evidence available to suggest that any of these risks have declined in recent years in parallel with changes in the tar/nicotine yields of cigarettes. Indeed there is a dearth of information on any possible relationship between yields and risks to the unborn or recently delivered child. This is an area which merits attention from researchers.

Conclusions

How far the total risk of premature death has been reduced by the smoking of lower tar/nicotine cigarettes is uncertain. A worthwhile reduction in the young smoker's risk of lung cancer has already occurred, which suggests that reductions will eventually appear throughout middle and old age. There is also an encouraging reduction in deaths from chronic obstructive lung disease which may, at least in part, be due to lower yields of tar and nicotine. However, there is no evidence that deaths from coronary heart disease, the major killer among smoking-related diseases, have been affected, and no evidence has been produced relating to risks to the children of smoking mothers.

It is debatable how much further this approach can proceed. In view of the discussion in Chapter 3 concerning the potential for tar as well as nicotine to cause cigarette dependence, any further lowering of tar delivery may simply lead to a compensatory increase in the amount smoked. Clearly more research is needed and preferably using prospective controlled trials, though these could be justified only in individuals who declared that they had no intention of stopping smoking [23] and who would be willing to smoke consistently cigarettes of measured tar/nicotine yield.

Whilst looking always for a government lead which will aim to encourage smokers to stop smoking altogether, a tar reduction programme should certainly be part of government strategy. Further reductions in the tar and nicotine deliveries of cigarettes could be made, and enforced, if necessary, by legislation.

References

1   US Department of Health, Education and Welfare. *Smoking and Health.* DHEW Publication No (PHS) 79-50066. 1979

2   Action on Smoking and Health. Pipe and cigar smoking. The report of an expert group appointed by Action on Smoking and Health. *Practitioner 1973; 210:* 645–648

3   Russell MAH, Jarvis MJ, Devitt G et al. Nicotine intake by snuff users. *Br Med J 1981; 283:* 814–817

4   Gori GB. Observed no-effect thresholds and the definition of less hazardous cigarettes. *J Environ Pathol Toxicol 1980; 3:* 203

5   Hoffman D, Tso TC, Gori GB. The less harmful cigarette. *Prev Med 1980; 9:* 287–296

6   Wald N, Doll R, Copeland G. Trends in tar, nicotine and carbon monoxide yields of UK cigarettes manufactured since 1934. *Br Med J 1981; 282:* 763–765

7   Fairweather FA, Carmichael BA, Phillips GF et al. Changes in the tar, nicotine and carbon monoxide yields of cigarettes sold in the United Kingdom. *Health Trends 1981; 13:* 77–81

8   Hammond EC, Garfinkel H, Seidman M et al. Tar and nicotine content of cigarette smoke in relation to death rates. *Environ Res 1976; 12:* 263–274

9   Wynder EL, Mabuchi K, Beattie EJ. The epidemiology of lung cancer: recent trends. *JAMA 1970; 213:* 2221–2228

10   Wynder EL, Stellman SD. Impact of long-term filter cigarette usage on lung and larynx cancer risk: a case-control study. *J Natl Cancer Inst 1979; 62:* 471

11 Kunze M, Vutuc C. Threshold of tar exposure. Analysis of smoking history of male lung cancer cases and controls. In Gori GB, Bock FG, eds. *Banbury Report 3 – A Safe Cigarette?* Cold Spring Harbour, New York: Cold Spring Harbour Laboratory. 1980: 251–260

12 Auerbach O, Hammond EC, Garfinkel L. Changes in bronchial epithelium in relation to cigarette smoking 1955–60 vs 1970–77. *N Engl J Med 1979; 300:* 381–386

13 Doll R, Peto R. *The Causes of Cancer.* Oxford: Oxford University Press. 1981

14 Higgenbottam T, Clark TJH, Shipley MJ et al. Lung function and symptoms of cigarette smokers related to tar yield and numbers of cigarettes smoked. *Lancet 1980; i:* 409–411

15 Shenker MB, Samet JM, Speizer FE. Effect of cigarette tar content and smoking habits on respiratory symptoms in women. *Am Rev Respir Dis 1982; 125:* 684–690

16 US Department of Health and Human Services. *The Health Consequences of Smoking. The Changing Cigarette: a Report to the Surgeon General.* Public Health Service, Office on Smoking and Health. 1981

17 Sparrow D, Stefos T, Bosse R, Weiss ST. The relationship of tar content to decline in pulmonary function in cigarette smokers. *Am Rev Respir Dis 1983; 127:* 56–58

18 Lee PN. Low tar cigarette smoking. *Lancet 1980; i:* 1365–1366

19 Wald NJ. Mortality from lung cancer and coronary heart disease in relation to change in smoking habits. *Lancet 1976; i:* 136–138

20 Castelli WP, Garrison RJ, Dawber TR et al. The filter cigarette and coronary heart disease: the Framingham Study. *Lancet 1981; ii:* 109–113

21 Kaufman DW, Helmrich SP, Rosenberg L et al. Nicotine and carbon monoxide content of cigarette smoke and the risk of myocardial infarction in young men. *N Engl J Med 1983; 308:* 409–413

22 Heller RF, Hayward D, Hobbs MST. Decline in rate of death from ischaemic heart disease in the United Kingdom. *Br Med J 1983; 286:* 260–262

23 Stepney R. Would a medium nicotine low-tar cigarette be less hazardous to health? *Br Med J 1981; 283:* 1292–1296

Chapter Ten

SMOKING IN DEVELOPING COUNTRIES

Previous College reports on smoking have been concerned almost exclusively with the problem of smoking and health in the United Kingdom. Smoking is, however, an international problem which has already begun to involve the developing countries. Many of these countries are burdening themselves with an avoidable epidemic which, in the absence of resolute action, will replace the problems of infectious and nutritional disease that are currently and rightly seen as public health priorities. This chapter does not seek to set out fully the extent of the smoking problem in developing countries: it aims rather to summarise outstanding features of the problem, to consider such action as is being taken, and to point out the dangers which lie ahead.

It should be recognised from the outset that the smoking problem in developing countries is linked inextricably to activities and attitudes in developed countries. Developed countries bear responsibility for demonstrating that firm action to reduce smoking is both necessary and feasible and for controlling the activities of multinational companies. The companies that dominate tobacco growing, manufacture, and sale in developing countries are all based in developed countries: indeed, three of the world's six largest non-governmental tobacco companies are based in the United Kingdom.

The stand adopted by the tobacco industry can be judged from a memorandum produced for the international tobacco industry after the Fourth World Conference on Smoking and Health in 1979, which included the following objectives [1]:

"We must try to stop the development towards a Third World commitment against tobacco.

We must try to get all or at least a substantial part of Third World countries committed to our cause.

We must try to influence official FAO and UNCTAD policy to take a pro-tobacco stand.

We must try to mitigate the impact of WHO by pushing them into a more objective and neutral position."

There can be no doubt that smoking in developing countries is an adversarial problem, and that only the most determined action by those concerned to promote health will succeed in curbing the activities of the international tobacco industry.

In many developed countries (including those in which the major multinational tobacco companies are based) certain forms of tobacco advertising and promotion have been restricted and levels of tar, nicotine and carbon monoxide in manufactured cigarettes have been reduced. Few such restraints apply in developing countries, where cigarettes are promoted in apparent disregard of their consequences for health.

The WHO Expert Committee on Smoking Control reported in 1979 that "failing immediate action, smoking diseases will appear in developing countries before communicable diseases and malnutrition have been controlled and that the gap between rich and poor countries will thus be further expanded." [2]. This development is already occurring, but international action or concern has not yet matched the scale of the problem.

TOBACCO CONSUMPTION IN DEVELOPING COUNTRIES

Precise information on tobacco consumption in developing countries is difficult to obtain. Sophisticated survey methods have for reasons of both expense and availability of suitable personnel not normally been introduced: much of the information available is therefore of a different nature from that obtainable in the United Kingdom. Those responsible for producing such information as is available are to be commended for their initiative, and it is to be hoped that international agencies such as the World Health Organization will promote further action to ensure provision and standardisation of appropriate data on smoking in developing countries. In the absence of good survey data in this area it will frequently be necessary to rely on information produced for and by commercial agencies.

Forecasts for the period 1980–85 show that the cigarette markets in developed countries are expected to produce a mean growth rate of

TABLE 10.1. Growth rates in cigarette markets in developed and developing countries 1975–80 [3]

Developed		Developing	
Austria	+ 1.8%	Brazil	+ 4.1%
Germany	+ 0.5%	Malaysia	+ 4.7%
USA	+ 0.5%	India	+ 5.6%
UK	– 1.8%	Venezuela	+ 5.6%
Belgium	– 5.3%	Pakistan	+ 6.1%

1.2 per cent, after which a decline is expected. Over the same period the anticipated Third World growth rate is 3.9 per cent. Figures for 1975–80 demonstrate the differences between selected developing and developed countries [3] (Table 10.1).

All available reports from developing countries indicate an increase in both the consumption of manufactured tobacco goods, and cigarette smoking in particular. In some cultures smoking amongst women is not yet common, while in others smoking amongst young people is apparently very rare, but overall trends in developing countries increasingly follow those in the United Kingdom and other countries where smoking has been an established habit for many years.

It has become almost commonplace to refer to the smoking problem in developing countries as 'tomorrow's epidemic' [4]. While much of the data collected from developing countries are not strictly comparable, some examples which indicate that smoking is already widespread in many such countries are listed in Table 10.2.

TABLE 10.2. Estimates of percentage of smokers of any form of tobacco product in rural and urban populations in various parts of the developing world

Place	% Adult Smokers			Reference
	Male	Female	Total	
Rural Katmandu	78.3	58.9	68.3	5
Urban Old Katmandu	64.6	14.2	37.0	5
Plains of Terai	60.7	48.4	54.7	5
Egypt: rural = urban	39.8	0.9	–	6
Lagos				
General	42.0	2.4	–	7
Medical students	72.0	22.0	–	8
Senegal				
Urban	80.0	–	–	7
Rural	15.0	–	–	7
Bangladesh				
Rural	67.0	1.0	–	9
Doctors	39.2	–	–	10
Brazil				
Rio de Sol province	–	–	38.5	11
Males (35–54 yrs)	62.8	–	–	11
Females (20–30 yrs)	–	33.0	–	11
China				
Urban Henan Province	56.0	1.0	–	12

Most surveys show a lower prevalence of smoking amongst females than in males, and a higher consumption of manufactured cigarettes in professional and office workers [13]. Regular smoking amongst children rose from six per cent at the age of 15 to 21.8 per cent at the age of 19 in Colombo, Sri Lanka [14], and was practised by 38 per cent of 18-year olds in Southern Brazil [11].

The smoking problem in developing countries is complicated by the existence of a variety of forms of traditional smoking materials. There is good evidence that these are harmful to health, sometimes in different respects to Western-style cigarettes. Despite the gradual switch to cigarettes, it is clear that the use of traditional smoking materials will continue for many years. Where there is a high incidence of smoking amongst women and in manual workers or peasants, the more traditional forms of smoking are more likely to be used [5] .*

TOBACCO AND DISEASE

While the bulk of evidence incriminating smoking as a unique and preventable cause of mortality and morbidity emanates from developed countries, there is an increasing body of evidence from the Third World to demonstrate that smoking is as harmful to health in developing as in developed countries. No governments or individuals concerned for the health of their communities should be misled into believing that further research on the health consequences of smoking is a necessary precursor to action.

The 1983 WHO Report [15] points out that lung cancer is already as common among cigarette smokers in developing as in developed countries [16,17]. Studies from India indicate that the relative risk for lung cancers in smokers is around 8.6 times that in non-smokers [18,19]. Deaths from lung cancer in Hong Kong men and women have been rising recently, and rates in women are among the highest in the world [17]. The incidence rates of lung cancer in the Natal Bantu are also very high for men, lying between those of the USA and those of England and Wales at 24 cases per 100,000 population. Lung cancer in men increased sixfold and in women about fivefold over an 11-year period [7].

Cancer of the oesophagus is more common in developing countries than in the developed ones. Tobacco consumption plays an important role in its causation [20], as is confirmed by studies from Sri Lanka [21,22], India [23,24] and Southern Africa [25,26]. The incidence of carcinoma of the oesophagus in blacks in Durban, South Africa and Zimbabwe is among the highest in the world, exceeded only by that in Turkmenistan, USSR [7]. Egyptian studies [27,28] confirm that the highest risk for bladder cancer is in cigarette smokers, particularly in association with schistosomiasis [28], and a similar association emerges in South African subjects [7].

Higher prevalence among smokers than non-smokers of non-cancerous

---

* These include: 1. The hookah (or hukka, goza, hubble-bubble); wet tobacco burned in an earthenware cup (chilum) and conveyed by pipes to water storage through which smoke passes before reaching the smoker. 2. The bidi (or biri); tobacco wrapped in leaf instead of paper. 3. Chutta (cigars prepared from home-cured tobacco); these are frequently smoked with the lighted end inside the mouth (reverse smoking). 4. Various forms of pipes. 5. Tobacco is also frequently chewed, sometimes in combination with other materials, such as lime, betel nut, or betel leaf, or taken in powdered form as snuff.

respiratory diseases is found in Singapore [29,30], India [31–34] and Nepal [35]. Although the relationship is sometimes less clear-cut when relatively small amounts of tobacco are smoked, studies from many other countries confirm the association. Reports from India [36], Africa [7] and China [37] confirm that smoking plays an important role in the development of cardiovascular diseases and to a lesser extent cerebrovascular diseases.

Investigations in developing countries confirm that tobacco consumption during pregnancy results in the birth of children with lower weight, and that peptic ulcer is also more common in smokers than in non-smokers.

It must be borne in mind that in some developing countries tobacco is smoked in traditional forms which may be even more noxious than manufactured cigarettes. The use of the bidi and the chutta has been much investigated in India. The bidi appears to produce as much tar as normally available cigarettes, often more [38], as well as posing an additional hazard. It must be smoked at a minimum rate of two puffs per minute (in order to keep it alight), as a result of which it may well be the most harmful form of all smoked tobacco [39].

Cancer of the mouth, one of the most extensively studied cancers in developing countries, has been especially associated with reverse smoking, where the lighted end is placed inside the mouth [22].

In addition to the effect of smoking alone, the effects of nutritional and infectious diseases common in developing countries will combine to amplify its harmful consequences. It may also be noted that in many developing countries average life expectancy is still relatively low, so that some of the diseases caused by smoking do not have time to develop. This will clearly change as countries become more affluent and start to resolve some of their other health problems.

SOCIO-ECONOMIC ASPECTS

Many developing countries are major tobacco growers. The Food and Agriculture Organisation (FAO) reports that tobacco is grown in about 120 countries and territories, the principal tobacco-producing countries being the People's Republic of China, the USA, India, Brazil, the USSR, Greece, Turkey, Japan, Bulgaria, Canada, the Republic of Korea and Zimbabwe. Tobacco is seen as a crop that can be grown relatively easily, on land that may be unsuitable for many other crops.

Tobacco in many developing countries is undoubtedly a major source of employment and cash income [40]. In Zimbabwe tobacco is the principal export earner [41] and the nation's largest employer of labour [40]. In Malawi, Tanzania, the south of Brazil and in the Indian state of Andhra Pradesh, tobacco provides a living for many thousands of farmers and other workers engaged in curing, packing and processing [40].

Regrettably, tobacco as a crop uses land that might otherwise have been available for more socially beneficial crops. It contributes to deforestation through use of wood for curing; contributes to employment problems by using labour intensively only at infrequent seasonal peaks; and provides economic benefit to only a very small number of individuals and companies. Whilst it is dangerous and short-sighted for a country to become economically dependent on a crop whose long-term future is bleak [41], nonetheless, it must be recognised that the short-term economic benefits are those of most immediate concern. Any attempts to control smoking in developing countries must recognise that health considerations are, tragically, likely to be perceived as both uncertain and long-term, whereas economic considerations are both short-term and readily apparent.

The international tobacco industry is to all intents and purposes controlled by six major corporations, which, together with state companies in countries where there is a monopoly (e.g. China, Japan), are responsible for the bulk of tobacco produced and consumed. The UNCTAD report on "Marketing and Distribution of Tobacco" [42] concludes: "Developing countries supply 55 per cent of world leaf tobacco through foreign controlled marketing channels; their processed exports are almost non-existent; they have no influence whatever in the design, output, and innovation of machinery; their aggregate receipts from the tobacco industry are based, almost exclusively, on the demand response and marketing decisions (of multinational tobacco corporations). . . ."

With their almost unprecedented concentration of financial power, technological know-how and productive capacity the tobacco corporations have become involved in all aspects of tobacco growing and production, from assistance to farmers to close liaison with governments [43]. The companies "operate in the Third World through a complex network of partnerships and licensing arrangements. Philip Morris International, for example, sells more than 175 brands in more than 160 countries and territories through 25 manufacturing and marketing affiliates, 18 licensees, and some regional export-sales organisations. The company's recent, rapid expansion in the Third World has been particularly striking. . ." [44].

The corporations are 'encouraged' by their home governments to promote tobacco growing and sales in the Third World. The United States until recently included tobacco in the "Food for Peace" programme of concessional agricultural sales to needy countries [44], while in the United Kingdom, Rothman International has been awarded the Queen's Award for Exports. In answer to a Parliamentary Question in 1979, the Government Minister responsible, Mr Douglas Hurd, stated that between 1974 and 1979, £119,000 had been given to Belize, and £67,000 to Malawi for the development of their tobacco industries, and a further £3,188,000 had been invested by the Commonwealth Development Corportion for this purpose in Malawi and Zambia [45].

The tobacco companies based in the United Kingdom are: British

American Tobacco, Rothman International, and the Imperial Group (which, for historical reasons, has no serious presence in the Third World). British American Tobacco is the world's largest tobacco company with, for example, 81 per cent of the market in Brazil and 39.8 per cent of the market in Indonesia [40]. BAT alone has 119 factories in 52 countries [40].

No major tobacco company has as yet accepted publicly that smoking is harmful to health; indeed, most of these companies avoid discussion of the evidence. For example, the Chairman of Rothman International, Sir David Nicholson (speaking as a Member of the European Parliament) said, "There is no medical evidence to prove that a few cigarettes, say ten to fifteen a day, are bad for you"; a publication of the Philip Morris company [46] starts, "Has it been established that smoking causes cancer and other diseases? No. . ."; and in a publication for employees produced by the British American Tobacco Company it is asserted that, ". . .although there is a statistical association between smoking and certain kinds of ill-health, it has not been proven that these illnesses are actually caused by smoking." While such an interpretation of the evidence will not deceive a well-informed public, the tragedy of developing countries is that the public there is not well-informed about the dangers of smoking. When short-term economic benefits are also seen to accrue from tobacco, denials of the evidence will often meet a sympathetic ear.

CONSTITUENTS

Information on the constituents of tobacco products in developing countries is scanty. From such information as is available, however, it is all too clear that cigarettes sold in developing countries have often been higher in average tar and nicotine yield than those sold in developed countries – not least in the host countries of the companies often responsible for their promotion and sale [47].

Information on tar yields produced for a UICC conference in the Philippines in 1976 is shown in Table 10.3 [4]. More recent information indicates that cigarette tar yields in the Philippines may not have been lowered: one current brand on sale produces 71mg tar. Tar yields for a range of popular cigarettes sold in the United Kingdom and in Australia in 1981 were in no case greater than 19mg tar per cigarette. By contrast these same cigarettes sold in Singapore gave tar yields of 19mg to 33mg per cigarette [48]. Even the brands with the lowest available tar yield would barely be described as 'middle tar' in the United Kingdom. In Thailand a sales-weighted average of 29.5mg tar is reported [3].

Tobacco companies claim that some reductions in tar and nicotine yield in developing countries are being made, despite at the same time denying the harmful consequences of smoking. For example, State Express King Size did yield 31mg tar and 2.0mg nicotine in Kenya [49].

TABLE 10.3. Brand yields of tar (mg/cigarette) in four countries: published in "Tomorrow's Epidemic" [4]

Brand	Philippines	UK	USA	Australia
Kent (BAT)	33	13	16.5	15
Kool	32	–	18	15
Marlboro (Philip Morris)	25	15	17	14
Chesterfield (Liggett & Myers)	31	16	19	18
Range of all cigarettes tested	24–44	4–34	2–31	5–22

1 Where there is more than one variety of the same brand, an average has been taken

2 'Low tar' brands have been excluded from the UK, USA and Australian figures

3 Cigarettes in the Philippines manufactured under licence by national companies associated with the brand owner

It now gives 16mg and 1.5mg nicotine, almost identical to the United Kingdom yields of the same cigarette. However, no comprehensive lists have been published which would allow an accurate appraisal of trends throughout the world.

It should be remembered that western named brand cigarettes do not often form a high proportion of cigarettes sold in developing countries. Thus even though reductions are made in tar yields, the overall impact is lessened by the sale of home produced, high tar cigarettes. Furthermore, some of the traditional smoking materials popular in developing countries also yield levels of tar, nicotine, and carbon monoxide well in excess of the average western-style cigarette, and pose added problems because of the vigorous inhalation necessary to keep the product burning.

ADVERTISING AND PROMOTION

Cigarettes are heavily advertised in developing countries in a manner that would be totally unacceptable in the countries where the companies producing them are based.

In countries where health education and awareness of the dangers of smoking are virtually non-existent, where adult literacy is low, where there is much less consumer advertising than in the West, and where the desire to copy western habits is all too apparent, even a relatively small expenditure on advertising can be effective, not least in simply promoting the idea and desirability of smoking.

Through much of the developing world cigarette advertising is blatant and forceful. Cigarettes are frequently advertised on radio and television at all times of day, on hoardings in remote areas and even on road signs. A leading cigarette brand in Africa is called 'Life', while in countries such as Egypt, Taiwan, Bangladesh, and Uganda names such as 'Cleopatra', 'Nefertiti', 'Long Life', 'New Paradise', 'Champion' and 'Sportsman' require little amplification. Advertising and promotional techniques ally the sophistication of the West to the smoking of cigarettes. Cigarettes are promoted as an essential adjunct to successful, healthy and glamorous living. Indeed in Kenya, where the market is growing by eight per cent per annum, the fastest growth rate is among educated 25–35-year old men of high income [50].

As in the developed countries smoking is promoted through sponsorship of sporting and cultural events. The most important sporting event in Africa (seen by an estimated 400 million people annually), the East African Safari Car Rally, is sponsored by Marlboro. Even in China, the booming Canton Trade Fair and a Grand Prix tennis tournament are sponsored by cigarette manufacturers [51].

A particular problem in developing countries is that cigarettes are frequently sold by the 'stick' (i.e. singly) often by children, for whom the cigarette thus appears at an early age to be an object of financial reward.

It is worth noting that while in developed countries the tobacco industry defends its advertising with the discredited argument that advertising is directed towards increasing brand-share, and not overall size of the market, in developing countries where the aim is even more clearly to encourage new smokers and existing smokers to smoke more, this argument is totally – and literally – incredible. For example, until the late 1970s one company, British American Tobacco, had a monopoly of the market in Kenya – yet was the country's fourth largest commercial advertiser [4].

THE ROLE OF THE TOBACCO INDUSTRY

Comment on the activities of the transnational tobacco corporations is almost nugatory. More than two decades after the first Report on Smoking and Health of the Royal College of Physicians [52], long after the evidence on smoking and disease has been clear beyond any responsible doubt, and in the face of resolutions from the World Health Assembly and many other prestigious national and international organisations, the international tobacco industry is attempting to ensure that as many people as possible take up this potentially lethal habit.

There can be no doubt that the tobacco industry should at the earliest possible opportunity cease all forms of advertising and promotion, and act to reduce the level of the smoking problem in developing countries. This may appear an unrealistic aspiration, but is no less than is demanded by the evidence.

ACTION TAKEN

Few developing countries have taken any serious action to control smoking. Perhaps they cannot in truth be blamed for this: the example set them by countries such as the United Kingdom — where the problem is even more urgent — is remarkably undistinguished.

Cigarette advertising has been banned in Mozambique, Jordan, Senegal, Afghanistan and Singapore, and is in theory restricted to some extent in Ecuador, Mexico, Panama, Paraguay, Egypt, Kuwait, Sri Lanka, Thailand and Malaysia [53]. Health warnings on packets or advertisements obtain in Bolivia, Brazil, Colombia, Costa Rica, Ecuador, Guatemala, Mexico, Panama, Peru, Egypt, Jordan, Kuwait, India, Sri Lanka, Thailand, Malaysia and Singapore [53]. Several developing countries have legislation restricting smoking in certain public places, but — as with legislation in other areas — this is not fully implemented. Product information (tar, nicotine) is required on packets in Ecuador and Egypt [6]. According to the WHO report on legislative action to control the world smoking epidemic, not a single developing country has introduced legislation to ban the sale of cigarettes to minors.

Valuable legislation has been introduced in Kuwait, Saudi Arabia and other Gulf States, where an upper limit of 15mg tar has been introduced alongside health education programmes and curbs on cigarette advertising, and in Egypt, where it is also illegal to import or export high tar cigarettes [6].

In developing countries, as in developed countries, when legislation is threatened the tobacco industry opposes any progress, and faced by possible defeat, offers instead of legislation a series of negotiated 'voluntary agreements'. Such agreements are invariably unsatisfactory, and are designed to avoid any effective action.

In few developing countries is there any serious health education on smoking — perhaps understandably, in view of more immediate health problems.

Some international organisations have made efforts to promote action on smoking in developing countries. The International Union against Cancer (UICC) has developed a programme on Smoking Control with the generous assistance of the Norwegian Government's International Aid agency, NORAD. The purpose of this programme is to generate national and regional activity through a series of reports [54], workshops, conferences, and site visits. The World Health Organization has already produced reports [47] and organised conferences and workshops, with the assistance of the Swedish Government Aid Organisation (SIDA). (As is noted above, the British Government has made no financial contribution to international smoking and health activity, but has given aid to tobacco manufacture in developing countries.)

Conclusions

It is almost unimaginable that at a time when major infectious diseases and malnutrition are potentially or actually conquerable, mankind should inflict upon itself a totally unnecessary epidemic of smoking-related diseases. Yet in the absence of firm action, cigarette smoking can be expected to spread at an increasing rate throughout the developing world. It is not possible at this stage to predict precisely the consequences of this increase, but it is certain that failing action to control smoking, its toll of avoidable death and disease in developing countries will far outnumber that in the less populous developed world.

Specific recommendations on advertising, reductions in tar yield, health warnings and education are listed at the end of this report. Ultimately, if no action is taken, the cost will be in lives. The international tobacco industry can be expected to oppose and hinder efforts to reduce smoking. In doing so it will be directly responsible for fostering the deaths of thousands, in the 20th century's most avoidable epidemic.

References

1   International Commission on Smoking Issues (ICOSI). *Internal memorandum 1979:* unpublished
2   WHO Expert Committee on Smoking Control. *Controlling the Smoking Epidemic. Tech Rep Ser No 636.* Geneva: WHO. 1979
3   World Development Movement. *Tobacco – A World Development Briefing.* 1982
4   Muller M. *Tobacco and the Third World: Tomorrow's Epidemic?* London: War on Want. 1978
5   Pandey MR. *Tobacco Smoking in Nepal:* unpublished
6   Omar MS. *Tobacco Smoking in Egypt:* unpublished
7   Taha A, Ball K. Smoking and Africa: the coming epidemic. *Br Med J 1980; 280:* 991–993
8   Elegbeleye OO, Femi-Pearse D. Incidence and variables contributing to onset of cigarette smoking among secondary school children and medical students in Lagos, Nigeria. *Br J Preventive and Social Med 1976; 30:* 66–70
9   Cohen N. Smoking, health and survival: prospects in Bangladesh. *Lancet 1981; i:* 1090–1092
10 Islam A. *Cigarette Smoking in Bangladesh. WHO Workshop on Smoking Issues.* Colombo: WHO. 1981
11 Achutte AC. *Tobacco Smoking Trends in Brazil:* unpublished
12 Weng, Xin-Zhi. *Tobacco Smoking Trends in China:* unpublished
13 Jayant K. *Tobacco Habits in Relation to Coronary Heart Disease. WHO Workshop on Smoking Issues.* Colombo: WHO. 1981
14 Karunaratne WA. *Tobacco Smoking in Sri Lanka. WHO Workshop on Smoking Issues.* Colombo: WHO. 1981
15 *Smoking Control Strategies in Developing Countries.* WHO. 1983: in press
16 Malik HK, Aileat BK. *Indian J Cancer 1976; 13:* 149–155
17 Chan WC, Colbourne MJ, Fung SC, Ho HC. Bronchial cancer in Hong Kong, 1976–1977. *Br J Cancer 1979; 39:* 182–192
18 Notwani PN, Rao N, Sirsat MV, Sanghvi LD. A study of lung cancer in relation to bidi smoking in different religious communities in Bombay. *Indian J Cancer 1977; 14:* 115–121
19 Jussawalla DJ, Jain DK. Lung cancer in Greater Bombay: correlations with religion and smoking habits. *Br J Cancer 1979; 40:* 437–438
20 Vutuc C, Kunze M. *Smoking and Diseases in Developing Countries.* Geneva: WHO. 1982
21 Stephen SJ, Uragoda CG. Some observations on oesophageal carcinoma in Ceylon, including its relationship to betel chewing. *Br J Cancer 1970; 24:* 11–15

22 Ganeshananthan N. Aetiological aspects of oesophageal carcinoma in Sri Lanka. *Ceylon Med J 1975; 20:* 3–19

23 Gangadharan P. Epidemiology of cancer of the oesophagus in India. *Indian J Surg 1974; 36:* 293–298

24 Reddy CRMM, Parameswari M, Rajakuman P, Yuchistaraneeju Y. Carcinoma of the oesophagus and its relation to smoking – an epidemiological assessment. *Clinician 1975; 39:* 136–142

25 Wapnick S, Castle W, Nicholls D et al. Cigarette smoking, alcohol and cancer of the oesophagus. *S Afr Med J 1972; 46:* 2023–2026

26 Bradshaw E, Schonland M. Smoking, drinking and oesophageal cancer in African males in Johannesburg, South Africa. *Br J Cancer 1974; 30(2):* 157–163

27 Makhyoun NA. Smoking and bladder cancer in Egypt. *Br J Cancer 1974; 30:* 577–581

28 Ibrahim AS, Omar MS. Schistosomiasis and tobacco as suspected risk factors in bladder cancer. *World Smoking and Health 1979; 4:* 38–42

29 Chew PK, Chia M, Chew SF et al. Asbestos workers in Singapore. A clinical, functional and radiological survey. *Arch Environ Health 1973; 26:* 290–293

30 Onn ZK, Kee CP. Ventilatory function in normal industrial Malay workers in Singapore. *Singapore Med J 1976; 17:* 242–247

31 Purohit CK, Sharma R. Chronic bronchitis in rural aged persons 60 years and above. *Indian J Med Sci 1974; 28:* 487–493

32 Radha TG, Gupta CK, Singh A, Mathur N. Chronic bronchitis in an urban locality of New Delhi – an epidemiological survey. *Indian J Med Res 1977; 66:* 273–385

33 Malik SK, Singh K. Smoking habits, chronic bronchitis and ventilatory function in rural males. *Indian J Chest Dis Allied Sci 1978; 20:* 73–79

34 Malik SK, Wahi PL. Prevalence of chronic bronchitis in a group of North Indian adults. *J Indian Med Assoc 1978; 70:* 6–8

35 Pandey MR. *Proceedings of the Tercentenary Congress of the Royal College of Physicians Edinburgh.* Edinburgh. 1981

36 Bordia A, Purbiya SL, Khabya BL et al. Comparative study of common modes of tobacco use in pulse, blood pressure, electrocardiogram and blood coagulability in patients with coronary artery disease. *J Assoc Physicians India 1977; 25:* 395–401

37 Wang KH, Liu KF. Hsi Yen Yu Kuan Hsin Ping Ti Kuan Hsi (An investigation on the relationship between smoking and coronary heart disease). *Chung Hua Hsin Hsueh Kuan Ping Tsa Chih 1979; 7:* 170–171

38 Hoffman D, Sanghvi LD, Wynder EL. Comparative chemical analysis of Indian bidi, and American cigarette smoke. *Indian J Cancer 1974; 14:* 49–53

39 Sanghvi LD, Jayant K, Pakhale SS. Tobacco use and cancer in India. *World Smoking and Health 1980; 5:* 4–10

40 *The Economic Significance of Tobacco.* Rome: Food and Agricultural Organisation. 1982

41 Gooch P. A future of challenges. *Tobacco Reporter; April 1982*

42 UNCTAD. *Marketing and Distribution of Tobacco. Report No TD/B/C.1/ 205.* Geneva: United Nations. 1978

43 *UN Publication No E.77 II D.7*

44 Eckholm. 4,000,000,000,000 cigarettes. *World Smoking and Health 1979; 4(2)*

45 Hansard 1979: 21 November: 421

46 Philip Morris. *What About Smoking and Health:* undated

47 *Smoking Control Strategies in Developing Countries.* WHO. 1983: In press

48 Singapore Government Statistics

49 Granada TV. *World in Action:* undated

50   Wickstrom B. *Cigarette Marketing in the Third World*. Gothenburg:
      University of Gothenburg. 1979
51   *Guardian; October 20 1980*
52   Royal College of Physicians of London. *Smoking and Health*. London:
      Pitman Medical. 1962
53   Roemer R. *Legislative Action to Combat the World Smoking Epidemic*.
      Geneva: WHO. 1982
54   Gray N, Daube M, eds. *Guidelines for Smoking Control, 2nd edition*.
      Geneva: International Union against Cancer. 1980

Chapter Eleven

HEALTH EDUCATION AND LEGISLATION

This chapter examines the effects of health education and legislation on the prevalence of smoking in the United Kingdom since 1960. It concludes that health education, in the broadest sense, has probably been responsible for the reduction in smoking that has occurred over the past two decades, but that legislation has been sadly lacking and voluntary agreements with the tobacco industry have been relatively ineffective.

In this chapter the term 'health education' includes all sources of information about the effects of smoking on health. Knowledge originating in scientific journals is gradually passed on to the public through a wide variety of channels, including the media, doctors, nurses, teachers and other professional and non-professional bodies. Through these channels, as well as through overt campaigns mounted by health education specialists, public knowledge of the hazards of smoking to health has steadily grown [1].

The aim of most health education is to reduce the prevalence of smoking; that is, by persuading smokers to give up completely and non-smokers never to start, to reduce the proportion of smokers in the population. Reduction in the number of cigarettes consumed by each individual smoker, though welcome, is not seen as the primary aim.

Data are available on prevalence and consumption from the General Household Survey (GHS) published by the Office of Population Censuses and Surveys biennially from 1972–82 [2] and from occasional National Opinion Poll Surveys [1] but in most detail from the Tobacco Research (now Advisory) Council [3]. Comprehensive data from 1956 were published in seven editions up until 1975 under the heading "Statistics of Smoking in the United Kingdom". Since then annual supplements have been produced by the industry, but not published. Data from this period have been made available to the College by the Tobacco Advisory Council and it is from this that Figures 11.1 and 11.2 have been prepared. It is seen that the percentage of current male smokers has steadily fallen from 75 per cent in 1956 to 50 per cent in 1981. In women prevalence remained static at 42–44 per cent from 1961–76, since when (as pointed out in Chapter 7) there has been a definite downward trend in the percentage of current female smokers. Because of the methods of sampling and analysis GHS figures are lower but show similar trends, prevalence falling in men between 1972 'and 1982 from 52 per cent to 38 per cent and in women from 41 per cent to 33 per cent.

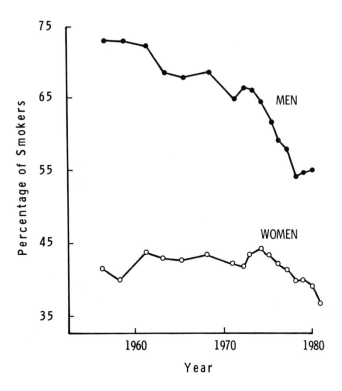

Figure 11.1. Prevalence of cigarette smoking in United Kingdom men and women from 1956 to 1981. Figures to 1975 published in [2], the Tobacco Research Council's statistical survey. Subequent unpublished figures reproduced from the Tobacco Advisory Council's data with permission

Consumption, on the other hand, has been more variable, though very recent trends are downwards. Male consumption assessed by manufactured cigarettes per head has fallen by 20 per cent since a peak in 1960. By the same index, smoking consumption in women peaked in 1974 but since then has begun to fall (Figure 11.2). GHS figures for 1972–82 fluctuate considerably but show no directional trend in men. In women consumption has been static since 1976.

Total tobacco sales reached a peak in the early 1960s, when in three years they exceeded 270 million pounds manufactured weight. Subsequently sales have been variable, but since 1974 have been consistently falling, reaching 226 million pounds in 1981.

Possible explanations for the recent falls in prevalence and total consumption include:

1. Economic factors, including changes both in the real price of cigarettes and in real disposable income;

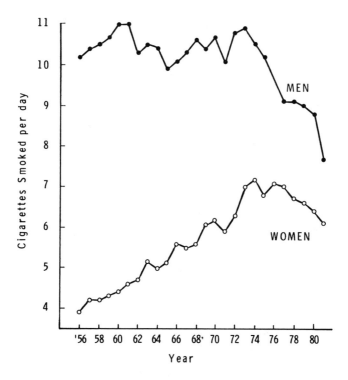

Figure 11.2. Average consumption of cigarettes per adult (men and women separately) whether smoker or not. Figure to 1975 published in reference 2, the Tobacco Research Council's statistical survey. Subsequent unpublished figures reproduced from the Tobacco Advisory Council's data with permission

2. The effects of a change in public attitudes to smoking unconnected with health education;

3. The effects of health education itself; and

4. The effects of legislation, and associated agreements.

These factors will be considered separately, though it is evident that they act together in various proportions to produce the observed changes.

Economic factors

It has been claimed that the price of tobacco cannot have played a significant part in the long-term decline in prevalence, because cigarettes were cheaper in real terms in 1980 than they were in 1960 [4]. Real disposable incomes also rose considerably during this period. However, a more detailed examination of the data shows that this is an over-simplification which hides a profound effect of price on tobacco consumption [5]. Consumption is determined on the one hand by the individual's need or desire for tobacco and on the other by economic factors. When desire or 'proclivity' is high, consumption is high and vice versa. Health education aims to reduce proclivity, and tobacco promotion to increase it. The economic attractiveness of tobacco is related to its price (which includes a variable proportion of tax) and an individual's real disposable income. Lloyd has calculated from available data that whilst it is true that there was a relative fall in tobacco price between 1961 and 1980, this was counterbalanced by a fall in proclivity so that consumption actually also fell [6]. Since 1980, the fall in the percentage of tax included in the price of tobacco goods has been reversed, and recent changes in consumption are related to economic factors. Estimates based on recent figures suggest that if the tax percentage on tobacco is kept at its present level, average consumption of cigarettes per head of population over 15 years of age is allowed to rise to maintain Government revenue from tobacco, then consumption would fall by 1999 to 30 per cent of present figures − just over two cigarettes per head per day.

Changes in public attitudes

Changes in attitudes towards smoking unconnected with health education might have played a part in producing some of the decline in smoking in recent years [7]. For example, smoking may have become unfashionable for reasons unconnected with the health risks. Little is known about such factors, but any effect has probably been small compared with the effects of health education.

HEALTH EDUCATION

Overall effects

The increasing weight of scientific evidence concerning the health risks of smoking first began to achieve prominence in about 1955. This was followed by the publication of the first Royal College of Physicians report in 1962, which was probably responsible for the sharp fall in both prevalence and consumption in 1962−3. Atkinson and Skegg [8], for example, suggest that it led to an immediate reduction of about five per cent in cigarette sales, although a slow recovery followed at the rate of one per cent per year; a similar fall and recovery occurred after the 1971 report [8].

The publication of the first Royal College of Physicians report, with the tremendous publicity it received, is a convenient point from which to date the start of serious anti-smoking education. The findings of the report were accepted by the Government, and the then Health Minister, Enoch Powell, asked local authorities to distribute posters and pamphlets publicising the harmful effects of smoking. Graphs and statistics featured in the report began to make their appearance in school textbooks, and numerous local initiatives followed, based on the report's recommendation. The report added impetus to moves which eventually resulted in the banning of direct cigarette advertising on television in 1965 and in the setting up of the Health Education Council (HEC) and the Scottish Health Education Unit in 1968. The second Royal College of Physicians report in 1971 was quickly followed by the College setting up the influential organisation Action on Smoking and Health (ASH).

About 20,000 copies of the first Royal College of Physicians report were circulated by the American Cancer Society to their members in the United States. This led inter alia to President Kennedy asking the Surgeon General to prepare a USA report. This was published in 1964 and led, as in the United Kingdom, to a sharp fall in smoking. Invoking the 'fairness doctrine' governing television advertising in the USA, health bodies were able to show one free anti-smoking advertisement for every four smoking ones. It was not long before the tobacco manufacturers willingly opted for a ban on television advertising as in the United Kingdom. During this period smoking declined steeply in the United States, though some resurgence has occurred since then [9].

In both Britian and the USA, though there has been a substantial fall in prevalence and also to a lesser extent in consumption, there is less certainty concerning how this has come about [10]. Evaluation of individual anti-smoking campaigns shows that none has ever produced more than a transient effect on smoking prevalence or consumption. Their value lies chiefly in drawing attention to the issue. Each initiative helps to reinforce the image of smoking as an undesirable habit, among both smokers and non-smokers. The mere association of the word 'clinic' with smoking implies that a once fashionable custom is now widely perceived as a condition requiring treatment. Further impetus is provided by the growing indictment of cigarettes as an environmental hazard. Whether or not passive smoking is harmful to the body, it is increasingly perceived as harmful to the rights of non-smokers. Supported by slogans such as the Scottish Health Education Group's (SHEG) "Smoking gets right up other people's noses", the growing demands for smoke-free air in public places have continued to weaken the image of smoking as a desirable habit. The subsequent restrictions on smoking in public may also have had a small but welcome effect on consumption.

In these circumstances, no single agency can be credited with the major share of responsibility for the success of the 'overall campaign'. Nevertheless, the entire movement was clearly initiated, and periodically revitalised, by the publication of the Royal College of Physicians reports, and, since 1971, has been energetically led by ASH. Major parts have also been played by the HEC and SHEG, supported by the Government Health Departments, and increasingly by the media companies.

Of the various national bodies, the activities of ASH, as the only specialist organisation, are worth considering in some detail. Through contact with politicians, civil servants and advertising control bodies, it has done much to counter the promotional activities of the tobacco companies. Perhaps its most appreciable contribution has been energetic support for the media. The continuous flow of accurate information and quotable comments from this source have gained thousands of column inches for the 'campaign' at minimum expense to the public purse. The greatest tribute to ASH's work has come from the tobacco industry, who found it necessary to subsidise a pro-smoking public relations campaign in the guise of a 'freedom movement' in 1979.

Specific campaigns

The most visible part of the anti-smoking campaign has been contributed by the HEC and SHEG in the form of mass media advertising and associated activities. These have included programmes intended to promote a healthy life-style in general, such as HEC's "Look After Yourself" and SHEG's "Dying Scotsman".

A more specific initiative designed for 7–11-year old children was attempted by HEC with the well-known "Superman" campaign (1980–83). This involved the use of the Superman character battling on television, the cinema, and in comics with a degenerate 'pusher' of cigarettes called Nick O'Teen. Particular efforts were made to involve children actively by inviting written requests for packs of material, including signed certificates testifying to their personal commitment against smoking. No fewer than 600,000 children wrote to the HEC as a result of the 1981 campaign, and considerable unsolicited publicity by the media was also obtained.

Widespread coverage was obtained by SHEG in 1982 with their sponsorship of the Scottish World Cup Football Team. The "Go for Goals" campaign based on the team's advocacy of non-smoking led to poster displays in every Scottish primary school; and similar coverage was achieved in Northern Ireland by the Ulster Cancer Foundation, the HEC and other organisations.

Evaluation of campaigns of this kind in terms of children's later smoking behaviour is not feasible, but the impact of the 1981 Superman campaign was still discernible one year later [11,12]. The mailing of Superman materials to primary and middle schools in Sheffield encouraged about 25 per cent of schools to devote additional time to anti-smoking education. Spin-off effects of such mass media campaigns could be of as much value as the direct effects of the campaign on its target audience. Though difficult to measure, indirect effects, for example an influence on parents or teachers, may be of great significance in the long run.

Specific quit-smoking campaigns for pregnant women by HEC and SHEG were carried out on several occasions in the 1970s. These generally produced a measurable but temporary effect on behaviour [13]. A general disappointment with the effects of anti-smoking advice for pregnant women has already been voiced earlier in this report (Chapter 7).

Besides the national health education agencies, major contributions have been made by the BBC and Independent Broadcasting companies. Numerous programmes on the harmful consequences of smoking have been broadcast. For example, the BBC with support from HEC, ASH and SHEG, put out a six-programme television series on smoking cessation in 1982. Watched by audiences of up to eight million, the series attracted considerable attention and led to requests for 120,000 leaflets. Evaluation revealed that the material was well received, and that cessation rates at three months were relatively high [14].

At a local level, health education officers (HEOs) employed by local health authorities have contributed to the overall campaign by initiating local smoking education programmes in schools, NHS premises and the workplace. In addition, two-thirds of the smoking withdrawal clinics in Britain are organised by HEOs. The number of clinics increased from about 20 in 1962 to 49 in 1980, though during this time several clinics closed whilst others started up.

The existence of these clinics has undoubtedly reinforced the overall campaign to tarnish the image of smoking, but their direct contribution to cessation rates has probably been rather small. Estimates give a success rate of only about 10—20 per cent at one year, so that the entire output for the 49 clinics operating in 1980 amounted to only about 350 ex-smokers [15].

In schools

The increasing contribution of HEOs to the work of other health and education professionals has probably been of much greater importance than their personal involvement with clinics. Instruction regarding the health hazards of smoking is now provided in secondary schools, though not necessarily for all pupils. It is also widely taught in schools as a component of general health education.

There are no baseline data from which to chart the gains in this field, but several indicators suggest that considerable progress has been made [16]. For example, national curriculum projects in health education were developed for the first time in the 1970s by the Schools Council and the HEC, often with support from SHEG. Six major projects containing materials relevant to smoking were published between 1977 and 1983. These have received an increasingly favourable reception from teachers, so that, for example, between 500,000 and one million children annually have been influenced by the Schools Council/HEC Health Education 5—13 Project and its associated television broadcasts. In addition, 15 per cent of all secondary schools had undertaken training in the use of the companion 13—18 project before its publication in 1982.

There has been growing support from local and national government.

Several education authorities (e.g. Devon and Calderdale) have required all schools to produce written policies for health education. Finally, the support of the Department of Education and Science in 1981 for health education as an 'essential constituent' in the school curriculum has given considerable impetus to the promotion of school health education [17].

Undoubtedly, therefore, even if there is no firm statistical evidence, the quantity of health education in schools has greatly increased. The same applies to quality. Recent approaches have included essentially factual projects involving a minimum of didactic instruction and a maximum of varied activity for the learner, e.g. the HEC/Sheffield Education Authority "My Body" Project and the Cancer Research Campaign's "Jimmy" Project in Glasgow, both for 10–12-year olds. For adolescents, projects have focused especially on attitudes to smoking rather than on simple transmission of information.

Evaluations of the "My Body" Project in Sheffield, have shown that its use leads to major gains in knowledge, favourable changes in attitudes [18], and a considerable influence on parents [19]. One independent cohort study in the Sheffield area has shown that the project produces a small, but statistically significant, reduction in the number of boys who try cigarettes [20]. Similar results, lasting for up to three years after the initial intervention, were obtained in an evaluation of the closely related "Berkely" or School Health Curriculum Project in the USA [21].

For teenagers, success in reducing recruitment to smoking has been claimed in the USA for a mixture of approaches, based on resisting the social pressures to smoke, and on the immediate, rather than the long-term physiological effects of smoking [22]. Accordingly, the HEC set up major projects in 1981 to investigate the acceptability of these techniques in British schools, and subsequently to evaluate their effectiveness in the prevention of smoking. Trials of a method involving the training of selected 12-year olds to lead group discussions [23] began in 25 local health and education authorities in 1982, and publications on the use of immediate physiological effects as a teaching method are in preparation. Hence schools are making a substantial and increasing contribution to education about smoking.

Adults

In 1981 ASH, HEC and SHEG produced "Give Up Smoking" (GUS) kits containing advice on giving up smoking in the form of a booklet, for use by general practitioners. The project was based on research by Russell [24], who obtained a five per cent success rate after one year (compared with 0.3% of unadvised controls). This appears to be cost-effective compared with smoking withdrawal clinics. More than one in three general practices (and almost three-quarters of all Scottish practices) asked for kits within six months of publication.

There has been less detailed evaluation of the contributions of other health professionals, but ASH, SHEG and HEC have all undertaken research and development projects in conjunction with nurses, health visitors, and midwives. Recognition by the nursing profession of the role of nurses, both as educators and examples, is being helped by the distribution of a variety of publications to support their work with patients and in the community. Publication of the ASH guide to Smoking Prevention in the NHS in 1981 provided a further stimulus to work on this topic. Efforts have been made by the Scottish branch of ASH to involve retail pharmacists in advising their customers about the hazards of smoking.

Smoking at work

There was little interest in this until recently. However, since smoking became a minority habit in about 1970, non-smokers have complained about their exposure to smoking at work with increasing frequency. A few companies have discouraged smoking at work, particularly in work space shared with non-smokers. Pressure on industry from national and local health organisations to formulate policies concerning smoking at work has increased. After several years, when there appeared to be little support from the Trade Unions, the 1981 Trades Union Congress approved a resolution forbidding smoking at the Annual Conference and called on all member Unions to "undertake a programme of education . . . on the dangers of smoking". The TUC has subsequently requested the HEC to join them in the preparation of a series of leaflets for working people on the hazards of smoking.

Efforts to promote cessation schemes in the workplace have also increased. These achieve similar success rates to non-industrial clinics [25], but attain much higher levels of participation among smokers, owing to their convenient setting.

Conclusions about effects of health education

Public knowledge about the risks of life and health that smokers run has steadily increased through many channels of information, but particularly through the media. As a consequence, increasing numbers of smokers have stopped and fewer children are starting to smoke.

But much ignorance remains. About 30 per cent of smokers deny that they risk harm in their health by smoking, and many who accept a possible risk consider it applies only to those who smoke more than they do. More serious is the fact that only a small proportion of those who accept any health risk realise that they could avoid it by stopping. More vigorous effort is needed to ensure that smokers do appreciate that even moderate smoking is dangerous and that the dangers can be avoided by giving up.

The overall climate of public opinion is probably the chief determinant of smoking behaviour in the community. The main obstacle to faster progress, therefore, lies in the existence of the 'anti-campaign', in the shape of cigarette advertising and sponsorship, costing about £100 million annually, against the £2.5 million estimated annual expenditure on smoking education by government agencies.

LEGISLATION AND VOLUNTARY RESTRICTIONS

No legislation on restricting smoking has been enacted in the United Kingdom except for constraints, largely ignored, on the sale of cigarettes to children. Instead, the British belief in the merits of persuasion has resulted in a number of voluntary agreements between successive Governments and industry, which have fallen far short of the achievements of legislation in other nations.

The development of restrictions in the United Kingdom has so far reached only the second of the three stages described by Roemer as characteristic of smoking control in industrial countries generally [26]. These are:

1. Legislation in the period from 1890 to 1960 to prohibit sales of tobacco to minors, and to prevent fires due to smoking in places where the public congregates;

2. Voluntary agreements with some legislation in the 1960s and early 1970s following the recognition of the health hazards of smoking and dealing with specific problems, such as the labelling of cigarette packages and advertising;

3. Beginning in 1975, the enactment of comprehensive legislation dealing with multiple facets of smoking amenable to legislation (as in Finland and Norway, but not yet in the United Kingdom).

Various types of restrictive measures are feasible, and should be combined in any comprehensive legislation on smoking:

a. controls on the product itself;

b. prohibitions on smoking in public places;

c. restrictions on sales;

d. restrictions on promotion;

e. taxation.

Control of tobacco production

A total ban on the growing or sale of tobacco is widely regarded as impracticable. There are no bans of this kind anywhere in the world at present. Arguably any such ban would result in the clandestine growing, distribution and consumption of tobacco as with marijuana. This might stimulate organised crime, on a scale similar to that triggered by the Volstead (or Prohibition) Act in the USA.

Controls on the quality of cigarettes may be achieved by imposing limits on the amounts of harmful substances, e.g. tar or nicotine. Reductions in tar yields have been achieved through differential taxation and voluntary agreements between the Government and the industry in the United Kingdom, and the reasons for believing these may be reducing the incidence of smoking-related diseases have already been discussed (Chapter 9).

Many health educators, however, believe that to condone the use of low tar cigarettes is disadvantageous in the long run. This is because smokers may equate 'low' with 'safe', and so feel no need to give up completely. The young may also start smoking for the same reason; indeed, low tar cigarettes are easier to smoke for the novice. In addition, promotion of 'less hazardous' smoking implies support for smoking as a habit, and so undermines the main objective of the anti-smoking movement, which is to reduce death and damage to health from smoking. For these reasons, leading British anti-smoking organisations (e.g. ASH and the HEC) do not support the public promotion of techniques for 'less hazardous' smoking.

Restrictions on smoking in public places

In the United Kingdom legilsation to prohibit smoking in certain types of factories has long been in force as a means of reducing fire risks — known to cause 20 per cent of all industrial fires in 1974 [27]. However, even essential restrictions of this type are not fully enforced.

The problem of passive smoking has been discussed in Chapter 8. In the United States the Department of Health, Education and Welfare has introduced regulations to protect its own non-smoking employees, and these regulations were adopted subsequently by all other Government agencies. They now provide that no worker be required to work in an atmosphere containing tobacco smoke, and this applies to conference rooms, classrooms and eating places. In Minnesota the Clean Indoor Air Act of 1975 goes still further, by permitting smoking only in private, enclosed offices occupied exclusively by smokers. In the United Kingdom there are no such wide reaching restrictions.

Special problems are found in hospitals. In Britain, some areas are non-smoking for reasons of hygiene (dispensaries, microbiological laboratories) and some for reasons of danger from explosion. Many hospitals impose bans in wards, corridors and lifts, and some have shown that the open ward system need not pose any problem. The DHSS has issued guidelines to hospital managers recommending that smoking by staff should be confined to specific areas. This is essential if the public is to be persuaded that smoking is no longer acceptable.

As highlighted in Chapter 6 on Children and Smoking, particular attention needs to be paid to smoking in schools. Despite the difficulties, legislation banning all smoking on school premises already exists in France, Finland, Italy and Bulgaria — though its enforcement may not yet be universal. In addition, sales of cigarettes in or near all educational establishments are prohibited in the USSR and Bulgaria.

Unlike the situation in the USA, where some 30 states have passed legislation restricting smoking in public places, no national restrictions or legislation yet exist in the United Kingdom concerning smoking in public. Though there has been an increase in non-smoking areas on public transport such as railways and subways, and in cinemas and other places of entertainment, there is much room for improvement. Smoking in restaurants still causes discomfort to non-smokers and few public houses make provision for non-smokers.

The non-smoking majority in the United Kingdom has every right to expect protection from the discomfort and danger of other people's cigarette smoke, as has already been largely achieved elsewhere. The most advanced legislation is found in Finland and Norway. The general approach in the Finnish Act has been described as 'rule-switching', i.e. smoking is prohibited unless specifically allowed [28].

Restrictions on sales

Since the repeal of the licensing laws relating to the retailing of cigarettes in 1963, there have been no restrictions on the sales of cigarettes generally in Britain. Ironically, sales in supermarkets were allowed shortly after the publication of the first Royal College of Physicians report. The reintroduction of licensing might be a useful first step towards restriction of sales to limited outlets, but would involve considerable additional bureaucracy.

The sale of cigarettes to children aged under 16 has been prohibited in Britain since 1908. Unfortunately, as ASH surveys in 1975 and 1981 showed, the law is very little observed by tobacconists [29]. In addition, the continuing existence of vending machines vitiates the residual effectiveness of this legislation. Fortunately, vending machines are generally being withdrawn, except from supervised locations, owing to vandalism and theft.

Restrictions on promotion

Under the 1964 Television Act a regulation was introduced in 1965 to ban the advertising of cigarettes on television. It was passed after a refusal by the tobacco industry to restrict advertising to the period after 9pm [30] and represents the only legislation in this area in the United Kingdom. A series of voluntary agreements concluded between the Department of Health and Social Security and the industry resulted, among other provisions, in an advertising code forbidding the association of cigarette brands with manliness, feminine allure and social, sexual, business or sporting success. In addition, advertising is not to appear in media directed to the young, nor must it persuade non-smokers to take up smoking. Regrettably, these guidelines are frequently flouted.

The 1980–2 voluntary agreement added further restrictions, including a ban on cigarette posters adjacent to schools and children's playgrounds; a 30 per cent reduction in the use of posters generally; and a ban on the advertising of high tar cigarettes. A wider variety of health warnings was also introduced. Similar, but scarcely stricter, restrictions were added in the 1982-4 agreement, and a single health warning was again adopted.

These restrictions on advertising have caused the tobacco companies to explore alternative methods of drawing attention to their products. This, in turn, has led to a considerable increase in sponsorship, especially of sporting events likely to be televised. Within just a three-week period recently, press coverage included Embassy sponsorship of darts, bowls and snooker, Benson and Hedges sponsorship of cricket, tennis and snooker, John Player of cricket, rugby and motor racing, State Express of rugby and tennis, Peter Stuyvesant of sailing and bobsleigh, and several others. Marlboro's move into Formula One racing is accompanied by publicity stating, "We are the number-one brand in the world. What we wanted was to promote a particular image of adventure, of courage, of virility" [31]. Such sentiments would not be allowed in direct advertising: in sports sponsorship the tobacco companies get away with it. Sadly basketball, which had at one time decided to refuse sponsorship from tobacco and 'hard liquor' companies, has had to reverse this decision because of lack of sponsorship from elsewhere.

Allied to their direct sponsorship of sporting activities is the recent development of sponsorship through book publications. The Macmillan and Silk Cut "Nautical Almanac" has reached three annual editions; now there is the same combination's "Ski Guide". Rothmans Publications have produced 13 editions of their "Football Yearbook" and now they have added "Rugby" and "Rugby League". Benson and Hedges have cornered the cricket market with their first "Cricket Year". For the tobacco manufacturer, books like these are relatively inexpensive compared with most advertising costs, tend not to be thrown away, and are a clever medium to maintain promotion as pressures on direct sponsorship of sporting events increase.

Voluntary agreements concerning sports sponsorship between the Government Department of Environment and the industry were concluded in 1978 and more recently in 1982 (to run until 1985). This later agreement required the inclusion of health warnings on advertisements associated with sponsored sporting events and forbade sponsorship where most participants are aged under 18, but was widely considered inadequate.

A further strategy is the use of cigarette brand names in the promotion of travel interests. Rothmans started the trend with Peter Stuyvesant Travel and now Gallagher have come up with Silk Cut Master Class holidays and Philip Morris with Marlboro Adventure holidays. Both Channel 4 and the "Standard" newspaper have featured Peter Stuyvesant Travel. Though the tobacco companies argue that "it is entirely reasonable for us to build independent new businesses" using brand names "recognized for their quality and reliability", this is clearly a subtle new form of indirect advertising. Add to all this the promotion of the theatre, opera and concerts and it is abundantly evident that the tobacco companies have opened up a wide range of options for keeping the smoking image in the public eye.

Taxation

As pointed out earlier, economic factors do play a significant role in cigarette consumption. The tax fraction in the price of cigarettes was close to 0.70 in the early 1960s but fell to 0.63 in 1973, since when there has been a steady return to 0.71. If the Exchequer had not allowed the tax fraction to fall — particularly from 1969 to 1973 — then an earlier and steeper decline in cigarette consumption would almost certainly have occurred. Whilst keeping the tax fraction constant will certainly reduce tax revenue as the effects of health education take effect, it is important to emphasise that only a relatively small increment in tax fraction, initially of around one per cent per annum, would be required to maintain Government revenue at its present level.

Effects of legislation and voluntary agreements

This list of restrictions may, superficially, appear impressive. In practice, their value in controlling smoking has probably been minimal.

The first objection to any form of tobacco promotion, whether through advertising or sponsorship, is that it promotes a climate of acceptability towards smoking. As we have already pointed out, the creation of a hostile climate of opinion is the most potent approach open to health educators. Continued tolerance for any form of promotion of smoking involves tacit acceptance that smoking is not a serious health hazard.

In the United Kingdom many smokers are known to consider that smoking cannot really be harmful because the Government continues to allow it to be, advertised. The health warnings intended to negate this impression are well known to be ineffectual [32], and are usually carefully 'designed out' of the main part of advertisements.

The industry defends its advertising on the grounds that it has no effect on the prevalence of smoking, but is simply concerned with maintaining brand loyalties. Its opponents believe that advertising creates additional demand for cigarettes, and may influence the young to take it up. In any case it is difficult to understand why cigarettes are advertised even in countries where a single company has a monopoly of sales, if maintaining brand loyalty is the only aim (see Chapter 10).

Nothing can detract, however, from the point that advertising maintains a favourable climate of opinion, and thereby negates the efforts of health educators. Though a complete ban on tobacco promotion might seem to have little immediate effect on prevalence or consumption, it would be very likely to lead to an acceleration in the current slow rate of decline of these figures within two or three years [33]. The experience in Norway and Finland, where all forms of advertising are forbidden, lends support to this hypothesis, especially so far as children are concerned.

An advertising ban was introduced in Norway in 1975 as part of a comprehensive programme designed to tackle the smoking problem. Whilst it is difficult, therefore, to single out the effects of this one aspect, it is one of the more striking, and controversial, aspects of their programme, and some conclusions about its effects can be drawn. First, per capita consumption of cigarettes by Norwegian adults (over 15 years) was steadily climbing until 1970, when the Act was first discussed in the Norwegian parliament, and since then first remained constant and is now falling (Figure 11.3). Secondly, from 1975, the date of the enforcement of the Norwegian "Act on Restrictive Measures for the Marketing of Tobacco Products", the percentage of male smokers

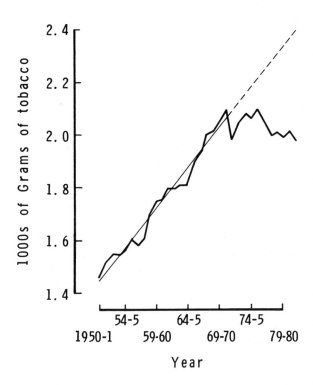

Figure 11.3. Consumption of cigarettes per adult per annum in Norway. In 1970 the Norwegian Tobacco Act, which included a ban on cigarette advertisement, was first discussed. In 1975 the Act became law. The dramatic change in consumption which occurred in the 1970s is clearly illustrated

has fallen from 52 per cent to 40 per cent, though there has been no change in the percentage of women smokers [34]. Finally, important information emerges about the uptake of smoking by children. In each of three age groups (13, 14 and 15 years) the percentage of smokers had been rising up until 1975. In 1980, five years after the advertising ban, the prevalence of smoking had fallen in each age group and in both sexes [34]. If an advertising ban affected only the uptake of smoking by children, the ultimate benefit to mankind would be enormous, and the importance of introducing legislation to enact such a ban cannot be over-emphasised.

In the field of sponsorship, present restrictions seem particularly feeble — no doubt stronger controls could not have formed the subject of a 'voluntary' agreement. At present, sponsorship of televised sports events helps to associate smoking with active, 'healthy' pursuits, and in effect, reinstates illegal cigarette advertising on television at minimal cost. It is particularly regrettable that the then Minister of Sport refused even to discuss restrictions on sports sponsorship with the Presidents of the Royal Colleges in 1981, despite the Government's acceptance of the health hazards of smoking. Sponsorship of cultural activities such as theatrical or operatic productions is probably undertaken for a different reason: to improve the industry's image with the decision makers. Efforts to close off these avenues of indirect advertising and brand name sponsorship are urgently required, for they directly negate the efforts of the health educators.

Not surprisingly, both the World Health Organization [35] and the United Kingdom Conference of Medical Royal Colleges [36] have called for the cessation of all forms of tobacco promotion.

Conclusions

As we have shown, much has been achieved by health education in the broadest sense in reducing the prevalence of smoking in the United Kingdom, at least among men. But little has been gained through legislation to date. Both of the laws in this field are either circumvented (advertising on television) or not enforced (sales to children).

As a result, a powerful pro-smoking campaign continues to flourish, and especially through sponsorship, seeks to maintain the acceptability of this dangerous addiction.

If the United Kingdom is to conform to the WHO appeal for "health for all by the year 2000", the single most effective step will be the adoption of a comprehensive policy for smoking control by all arms of Government, both national and local.

The drawing up of a comprehensive Government tobacco control policy, starting with the banning of all forms of promotion, could take advantage of the growing disfavour seen in public attitudes towards smoking, to bring about a dramatic fall in smoking prevalence in this country.

References

1   NOP Market Research Limited. *Random Omnibus Survey Carried Out for the Office of Population Censuses and Surveys on Smoking Habits.* London: OPCS. 1981
2   Office of Population Censuses and Surveys. General household survey: cigarette smoking 1972 to 1982. *Government Statistical Service GHC 83/2 July 1983*
3   Tobacco Research Council. Lee PN, ed. *Statistics of Smoking in the United Kingdom. With unpublished supplements (1977–82).* 1976
4   Smoking and how to stop. *Which 1980; August:* 473–477
5   Sinnott PRJ, Gillian RJ, Kyle PW. *The Relationship between Total Cigarette Consumption in the UK.* London: Metra Consulting Group Limited. 1979
6   Lloyd BB. *Personal communication 1983*
7   Capell PJ. Trends in cigarette smoking in the United Kingdom. *Health Trends 1978; 10:* 49–54
8   Atkinson AB, Skegg JL. Control of smoking and price of cigarettes – a comment. *Br J Preventive and Social Med 1974; 28:* 45–48
9   Warner KE. The effects of the anti-smoking campaign on cigarette consumption. *Am J Public Health 1977; 67:* 645–650
10 Leventhal H, Cleary PD. The smoking problem: a review of the research and theory in behavioural risk modification. *Psychol Bull 1980; 88:* 370–405
11 Cocks, Williams Associates. *Evaluation of the Superman campaign 1982. Report to the Health Education Council*
12 Wilcox JS. *Evaluation of the HEC Superman campaign in Sheffield primary and middle schools 1981. Report to the Health Education Council*
13 Henderson RS. *A Report for the Scottish Health Education Unit as a Result of Smoking in Pregnancy Programme Evaluation over a Five Year Period 1975–80.* Glasgow: University of Strathclyde. 1980
14 Moreton WJ, East R. *Evaluation of the BBC Smoking Cessation Series, So You Want to Stop Smoking.* Kingston: Kingston Polytechnic: in press
15 Raw M. *A Brief Guide to the Smoking Treatment Literature.* London: Action on Smoking and Health. 1982
16 Reid DJ. Into the mainstream. *Times Educational Supplement 1981; 17 April:* 21
17 Department of Education and Science. *The School Curriculum.* London: HMSO. 1981: 7–8
18 Wilcox B, Engel E, Reid DJ. Smoking education in children: UK trials of an international project. *Int J Health Educ 1978; 21:* 236
19 Wilcox B, Gillies P, Wilcox JS, Reid DJ. Do children influence their parents' smoking? *Health Education J 1981; 40:* 5–10
20 Wilcox B, Gillies PA. *A Longitudinal Cohort Study of the Effectiveness of the My Body Project. Report to the Health Education Council 1981*
21 Milne AM, Marshall-Mies J, Colmen JG. *A Study of Impact of the School Health Curriculum Project on Knowledge, Attitude and Behaviour of Teenage Students.* Washington DC: Center for Disease Control's Bureau of Health Education. 1975
22 Evans RI, Rozella RM, Maxwell SE et al. Social modelling films to deter smoking in adolescents. *J Appl Psychol 1981; 66:* No 4
23 Arkin RM, Roemhild HE, Johnson CA et al. The Minnesota smoking prevention program. *J Sch Health 1981; 51 No.9:* 611–616
24 Russell MAH, Wilson C, Taylor C, Baker CD. Effect of general practitioners' advice against smoking. *Br Med J 1979; 2:* 231–235
25 Moreton WJ, East R. *Smoking Cessation Programmes in the Workplace.* Kingston: Kingston Polytechnic: in press
26 Roemer R. *Legislative Action to Combat the World Smoking Epidemic.* Geneva: WHO. 1982

27   Olsen DVL. *The Cost of Smoking to Industry.* Belfast: Ulster Cancer Foundation and ASH. 1981: 18

28   Rimpela M. *Experience with the Finnish Anti-smoking Programme.* Helsinki: National Board of Health, Office of Education. 1982

29   Action on Smoking and Health. *Surveys on the Sale of Cigarettes to Children.* London: ASH. 1975 and 1981

30   Marks L. Policies and postures in smoking control. *Br Med J 1982: 284:* 391

31   The Sponsors' Racing Formula. *Newsweek 1983; March 21*

32   Herail RJ, Lovatt EA. Why anti-smoking advertising loses out. *World Medicine 1979; 14:* 15–17

33   Hoffman WE. The impact of tobacco advertising and promotion of cigarette consumption. In Ramstrom LM, ed. *The Smoking Epidemic, a Matter of Worldwide Concern. Proceedings of the Fourth World Conference on Smoking and Health.* Stockholm: Almqvist and Wiksell. 1979

34   Bjartveit K, Lochsen M, Aaro E. Controlling the epidemic: legislation and restrictive measures. *Can J Public Health 1981; 72 Part 6:* 406–412

35   World Health Organization. *Controlling the Smoking Epidemic: Report of the WHO Expert Committee on Smoking Control. WHO Tech Rep Ser 636.* Geneva: WHO. 1979

36   Medical News Report. Call for stronger government action against smoking. *Br Med J 1980; 281:* 1574

Chapter Twelve

RECOMMENDATIONS

Each of the previous College reports has concluded with a list of recommendations for action. Sadly, through apathy and vested interests, very few of these have been adopted. That is no reason for us to fail to make similar recommendations again. The health risks of smoking do not lessen with the passage of years, rather they increase. As more and more suffer the consequences of this unnecessary habit the urgency for action remains as strong as ever.

Action to control and eventually abolish the distress caused by smoking-related diseases and the burden they place on the National Health Service has to be taken by smokers, by non-smokers, by educators both in school and beyond, by health care professionals and, most importantly, by the Government.

ACTION BY SMOKERS

Smokers are responsible for their own health as well as for that of those about them, yet most are still unaware of the grave dangers of smoking or of how they could avoid them.

Most think that only those who smoke heavily (by which they mean those who smoke more cigarettes than they do themselves) are likely to get serious illnesses caused by smoking. In fact about one-third of all premature deaths caused by smoking occur in smokers of fewer than 20 cigarettes per day. Many smokers think that only those with 'weak lungs' run any danger of serious illness because of their smoking. In fact (as shown in Chapter 5) it is almost impossible to tell in advance which smokers are going to be cut down by their smoking. Few smokers realise that about one in four of them will be killed by smoking and that, on average, a smoker of 20 cigarettes a day will lose about five or six years of life. Nor do they realise that the dangers of smoking are greatly reduced by stopping. The increasing likelihood of death from lung cancer with advancing age stops when smoking ceases, and the risk declines to a level close to that of the non-smoker after 10 years free from exposure to cigarette smoke (Chapter 3). Deaths from coronary heart disease are reduced by two-thirds in the first two years after stopping smoking (Chapter 4), and the decline of the victim of chronic lung disease into a state of irreversible disability can be halted (Chapter 3).

Finally, few smokers are aware of the harm they may do to others. A mother who smokes inflicts harm on her unborn child; parents who smoke both impair the health of their children by polluting the air they breathe and, by their example, encourage them to damage their own health by taking up smoking. A husband who smokes may increase his wife's risk of lung cancer, and presumably a wife does the same to her husband. Breathing other people's smoke is not merely very unpleasant, it can also be harmful (Chapter 8).

Smokers who accept the harm that smoking does to them will wish to stop. The committee recognises that for the regular smokers this is no easy achievement. Though 70 per cent of smokers may try to give up, only some 20 per cent at present succeed, and women find it especially difficult (Chapter 7). Most people who have stopped have done so with little or no specialist help. Many aids are, however, available and a summary of the committee's advice to smokers wanting to give up will be found in the Appendix.

Smokers who cannot or do not wish to stop often switch to a brand with a lower tar and/or nicotine delivery.* It is important to summarise here the evidence detailed in Chapter 9 that such cigarettes are less harmful. The lung cancer risk does seem to be reduced substantially and there is a suggestion of a fall in the risk of death due to chronic obstructive lung disease. However, there is no evidence that the smoking of cigarettes of reduced tar or nicotine yield reduces deaths from coronary heart disease – which numerically is the greatest killer amongst the smoking-related disorders. Furthermore, it is possible to change to a cigarette of lower tar or nicotine yield which has a higher yield of carbon monoxide. This could be especially harmful to elderly smokers with heart disease or in pregnant mothers.

The committee must emphasise that the only sure way to halt the rising death toll from smoking is for more smokers to stop. For smokers who cannot give up the habit, a less dangerous form of cigarette should be used. Reductions in cigarette tar yields seem to have produced most effect, and a cigarette which maintained a reasonable yield of nicotine would probably be more likely to satisfy the addict. But no such cigarette can be regarded as safe. Switching to cigars or a pipe will reduce the risk only if the inhaling habits of smoking, characteristic of the cigarette smoker, can be broken.

ACTION BY NON-SMOKERS

Those who do not smoke should continue to press for further restrictions on smoking, both at home and in public places. In their homes they can ask visitors not to smoke, or, as many now are beginning to do, display non-smoking notices. In restaurants they can urge proprietors to confine smoking to a designated area, pointing out their preference for eating in an atmosphere which is clear of smoke. Non-smoking should become an accepted rule on public transport. At work non-smokers should demand freedom from a smoke-polluted

* Copies of the DHSS list of yields of cigarettes can be obtained from Health Authorities and are often posted in Chest Clinics and doctors' surgeries.

atmosphere. The more firmly non-smokers speak up for their right to breathe smoke-free air, the more rapidly will adequate provision be made for their convenience and protection.

Policies on smoking in public places should take account of the fact that now smokers are in a minority. The aim must be to create a society in which non-smoking is the norm, with smoking areas designated where necessary and convenient, rather than the reverse, as at present.

EDUCATION

Teachers have a special responsibility for reducing the numbers of children who start smoking. A good example by teachers is essential. No teacher should smoke on school premises. Even if teachers dismiss the risk to themselves they must realise that smoking in school encourages pupils to follow their example and thus to incur life-long risks which, if they appreciated them, they might not wish to run.

Teachers should give urgent attention to ways by which they can bring education on healthy habits into a central position in the curriculum. A wide variety of health instruction programmes are now available and in use (Chapter 11). It is vital that they are properly evaluated. To succeed they must be based on a thorough understanding of the factors which encourage children to smoke, on planned involvement by parents and on giving realistic advice which equips children to resist peer pressure to smoke (Chapter 6).

Education outside school falls within the province of the communicators in society — those in television, in journalism and in advertising. There has been a welcome upsurge in the use of imaginative techniques, particularly on television, which educate the public about the health risks of smoking. The skills so obvious in commercial advertising can and are being harnessed for anti-smoking campaigns. The wide impact of television documentaries was exemplified by the wave of public horror that followed the featuring of illness and death due to asbestos exposure, a hazard which is responsible for a minute number of deaths when compared with those due to smoking.

Women need advice and help about smoking, perhaps even more than men. They have special problems in relation to smoking during pregnancy and whilst taking the contraceptive pill (Chapter 7). They find giving up smoking much more difficult than men do. Women read magazines widely and a concerted campaign about the dangers of smoking through women's magazines would be of enormous benefit.

THE HEALTH CARE PROFESSIONS

The greatest responsibility and potential for action and example still lie with workers in the health care professions. Doctors must unflinchingly maintain their stand against smoking. They have special opportunities for giving advice, for they encounter many smokers who during an illness are often ready to stop smoking. Most consultations between a doctor and his patients can be used as occasions for explaining the dangers of smoking. Equal responsibility is shared by all those who work in health care, particularly nurses and medical students. Health care workers have an obligation not to smoke themselves and, particularly, never to smoke in the presence of patients. It is regrettable that it is still necessary to reiterate the recommendations put forward in the last College report (1977) that there should be no smoking at meetings of committees concerned with health care services, and that tobacco should not be sold in hospitals or other health care premises.

Control of smoking within hospitals could be far stricter. A no-smoking rule can be enforced without objection and even welcomed in acute general medical and surgical wards. Co-operation between medical, nursing and ancillary staff is essential to ensure that no staff member is ever seen to be smoking on the ward itself or in the side rooms. Within this overall strategy compassionate consideration must be shown to long-term psychiatric or geriatric patients and to the dying.

The profession has not taken sufficiently seriously the problem of the smoker who wants to stop but is unable to do so. Despite an increase in activity recently, research has not yet led to a reliable stop-smoking technique. Much further endeavour is needed to unravel the complex nature of addiction to smoking and the consequent difficulties in breaking the habit. Special attention needs to be given within the profession to the smoking problems of nurses under stress.

ACTION BY GOVERNMENT

Heavy responsibility rests on the Government for fiscal and legal measures which could lessen the impact of the smoking epidemic on the health of the nation. Since the Royal College of Physicians first reported on the vast dimensions of the burden of disease caused by smoking, successive Governments have shown regrettable unwillingness to take the sort of action which might at first contain, and ultimately overcome, the tragic consequences of smoking. What has been done is but a small measure of what could have been achieved. Certainly the Health Education Council was started and, with Government encouragement, it has spent more on public education about smoking than on any other health topic. But their budget for this purpose has been miniscule in comparison with the £50–100 million spent each year by the tobacco manufacturers on advertising. The worst aspects of this advertising were at first tempered by a voluntary agreement with the manufacturers. Frequent breaches of this voluntary code led to stricter monitoring by the Advertising Standards Authority, but the ingenuity of the manufacturers' advertisements has enabled forceful pro-smoking propaganda to continue, particularly through sports and cultural sponsorship. The Government has insisted on warnings being placed on cigarette packets (but never in effective terms nor in a prominent position) and on advertisements (but not so as to compete with the message of the advertisement). Besides these concessions the three most important recommendations which have been made in successive reports by the Royal College of Physicians, by ASH and by the Health Education Council have been firmly resisted. These are:

1 A ban on sales-promotion of tobacco

Apart from the effects of intense lobbying by the tobacco industry, resistance to such legislation seems to stem from the view that it would be 'wrong' to forbid sales-promotion of any goods which can be legally sold. This strange commercial ethic has no basis other than perverted logic and no such ethical dilemma has affected other countries which have banned tobacco advertising, and found it effective in reducing tobacco consumption (Chapter 11).

The tobacco manufacturers urge that their advertisements only affect brand loyalty and do not encourage smoking, yet they continue to advertise widely in countries where one company has a monopoly of sales (Chapter 10).

The only other possible reason for the Government's failure to ban promotion of such harmful goods as cigarettes may be fear of unemployment consequent upon a gradual decline of the tobacco industry.

Whatever measures might be taken to restrict sales promotion could, however, only have a gradual effect. There would be no sudden loss of jobs in tobacco manufacture, giving time for alternative employment to become available and for diversification within affected companies.

2 A steady annual increase in tax to keep the price of tobacco rising faster than the rate of inflation

It may seem strange that the Treasury should resist this most effective change, which would, at least in the short term, increase revenue. Because of their habituation many smokers would continue to buy increasingly expensive cigarettes. The Treasury would be able to accommodate to the long-term decline in overall tax revenue from tobacco by the gradual introduction of other fiscal measures (Chapter 11).

3 Reduction in tar, nicotine and carbon monoxide yields in cigarettes

The evidence that a universal reduction of the tar and nicotine yields of cigarettes would reduce the incidence of lung cancer is now clear enough to justify a firm policy in this regard. It is less certain what influence this reduction would have on other respiratory or on cardiovascular illnesses, but present evidence suggests that it would not be adverse and might be beneficial. The Government should aim to reduce the maximum yields per cigarette below 15mg for tar, 10mg for carbon monoxide and 1mg for nicotine as soon as possible. The Government should confer with tobacco manufacturers to see by what means and how rapidly this change could be brought about with and without the use of tobacco substitutes. They should then introduce legislation to ensure that the reduction is carried out over the agreed period. Meanwhile a tax differential between higher and lower tar/nicotine/carbon monoxide cigarettes could encourage the necessary trend.

A major reason for the failures of successive Governments to take effective action on smoking-related diseases is that they have lacked a co-ordinated approach to the different aspects of the problem. Since it is primarily one of disease control it is natural that the Department of Health should have a leading role, but the necessary changes of taxation, in industry (restrictions of smoking at work, redeployment), control of tobacco sponsorship in the arts and in sport, and provision of more time and money for health education in schools concern other departments. A co-ordinated policy between departments is surely needed, as is recommended in the report of the WHO Expert Committee on Smoking and its Effects on Health. It is this that has enabled Norway and Finland to produce their overall policies which are already having a notable effect on reducing smoking in those countries. Curtailment of smoking must be an essential part of the policy of any government sincerely concerned with the health of the people it serves, and such a policy demands a co-ordinated, interdepartmental approach.

The British Government – in common with all governments in developed countries – has a responsibility to control smoking, not only out of concern for the health of its own people, but in full awareness of its exemplary role towards developing countries (Chapter 10). Britain should encourage developing countries to ban all forms of advertising promotion for tobacco, to introduce clear, effective health warnings on cigarette packets and to develop health education programmes on smoking. In conjunction with foreign governments it could devise plans to provide alternative uses for land currently used for tobacco cultivation, and to retrain tobacco workers.

There is probably little that we can say to the multi-national tobacco companies that would not fall on deaf ears. We hope that they will read this report and at least accept that the grave concern within the medical profession about the enormity of the health problem presented by smoking has an unchallengeable basis in fact, and that they will take especial note of the criticism we level at their activities in developing countries.

Finally, there is a continuing need for research. Fields of particular importance include:

a)   renewed research into the components of cigarette smoke responsible for cardiovascular disease (Chapter 3)

b)   further exploration of factors which might influence susceptibility to the harmful effects of cigarette smoke and especially the potential influence of vitamin A on lung cancer risk (Chapter 5)

c)   the development of accurate measures of passive smoking and the consideration of what sort of large prospective studies could be designed to clarify the risks of smoking-related diseases in passive smokers (Chapter 8)

d)   further studies of the potential benefit of reduced tar/nicotine/ carbon monoxide yields in cigarettes, preferably using prospective controlled trials in smokers who are unwilling to give up cigarettes. In particular there is urgent need for direct evidence as to the effects of cigarettes delivering small amounts of everything except nicotine (Chapters 2 and 9)

e)   a thorough appraisal of existing health education programmes and the devising of new approaches based on recent knowledge of the factors which lead children to take up smoking and encourage them to persist with the habit (Chapter 6)

f)   much more research into the nature of tobacco addiction with the hopeful consequence of an increased understanding of how to overcome the difficulties certain smokers, especially women, have in stopping, even though they wish to do so (Chapters 2 and 7)

g)   a continued search for alternative aids for helping smokers to stop with proper scientific appraisal of their efficacy.

Appendix

GIVING UP SMOKING

There is no wonder cure for the smoker who wishes to give up. For some it is apparently easy, for others exceedingly difficult – but many thousands have given up, and done so with little or no medical or specialist help. Indeed, it is now true that a majority of people do not smoke, and find it easy to live without cigarettes.

The bedrock on which any plan to stop smoking must be based is your decision that you no longer wish to smoke. You may have been impressed by the long catalogue of health risks to smokers given in this report and elsewhere; you may be feeling guilty about the health risks you are imposing on others, especially if you are a pregnant mother; you may have been shocked by your own declining health; or it may simply be a question of cost. For whatever reason, you personally must have arrived at a point where you have made for yourself the decision that smoking will cease to be part of your life.

What do you do next? Plan a campaign. It may help to make a note of your personal pattern of smoking. Do you smoke just with friends, just at the office, only at home, only with meals? Recording when you smoke will help you to plan resistance to the craving for a cigarette at these times. Set a target date perhaps two or three weeks hence when you are going to become a non-smoker. It may be helpful to choose a relatively non-stressful time, such as a holiday or some other occasion when you can change your routine. You may be the sort of person who can do it all on your own. Most smokers gain help by telling their friends or, better, bargain to stop *with* a friend. It is more difficult to start again when every one knows you have made the decision to stop.

Stopping abruptly is probably more likely to be successful than cutting down. Heavy smokers may find a period of gradual reduction helpful before an abrupt stop. If you do choose to go the whole way by gradual steps, be very strict with yourself. Cut out cigarettes at specific times; ration the number you have available for each day. Do not attempt the 'saturation' method (smoking many times your usual number of cigarettes until you are literally sick of them) without medical advice: it can be dangerous.

Once you have passed zero day and actually stopped, you will need to keep a careful eye on those danger times in the day when you previously had a cigarette. Do not have any cigarettes in the house, watch out for meal times. Avoid meeting friends who are smokers. Travel in non-smoking compartments. Avoid at all costs that 'odd one'. It will grow into just another and another . . . . Reinforce your resolve by getting hold of literature about smoking from your doctor or from the Health

Education Council. Find other ways of coping with tension that do not rely on smoking a cigarette. Relaxation may be the way for you; on the other hand, exercise may be the answer. Sedatives and tranquillisers are of little use. Watch your weight; not because any increase is likely to harm your health but it may damage your self-image. Some smokers do put on weight after stopping smoking, but with a little care about diet, this settles down in due course to near normal again.

There are special aids: group therapy, snuff, graded cigarette holders, hypnosis, acupuncture and nicotine chewing gum. None of them has a very high success rate and, apart from nicotine gum, no one emerges as strikingly more effective than any other. Nicotine chewing gum, when used casually without special attention to technique, has proved no better than other aids, but if used carefully as recommended it has been found to achieve higher success rates. All of these aids are capable of helping some smokers, but none is a substitute for the will and resolve of the individual to give up.

Many who give up for a few days find they cannot resist any longer and are soon back smoking regularly again. This is inevitable with an addiction such as smoking. Do not let it damage your ultimate determination to give up eventually. Try one of the aids if you have not already done so; or change to another. You will eventually succeed if you really want to.

The longer you manage without cigarettes, the easier it becomes, and the more similar are your risks to those of people who have never smoked. Success in giving up breeds success. Your example will encourage other adults to try. As more adults do not smoke, fewer children will start what becomes a fatal habit to so many.

Finally remember changing to lower tar brands is no substitute for stopping. Even changing to a pipe or cigars it not without a risk. It is best to be a non-smoker.